T0144850

BASIC HEALTH PUBLICATIONS USER'S GUIDE

TO EASING MENOPAUSE SYMPTOMS NATURALLY

Learn How to Prevent Hot Flashes and Other Symtoms Safely and Naturally.

CYNTHIA M. WATSON, M.D.

JACK CHALLEM Series Editor

The information contained in this book is based upon the research and personal and professional experiences of the author. It is not intended as a substitute for consulting with your physician or other healthcare provider. Any attempt to diagnose and treat an illness should be done under the direction of a healthcare professional.

The publisher does not advocate the use of any partic ular healthcare protocol but believes the information in this book should be available to the public. The publisher and author are not responsible for any adverse effects or consequences resulting from the use of the suggestions, preparations, or procedures discussed in this book. Should the reader have any questions concerning the appropriateness of any procedures or preparations mentioned, the author and the publisher strongly suggest consulting a professional healthcare advisor.

Series Editor: Jack Challem
Editor: Laura Jorstad
Typesetter: Gary A. Rosenberg
Series Cover Designer: Mike Stromberg

Basic Health Publications User's Guides are published by Basic Health Publications, Inc.

CONTENTS

INTRODUCTION

If you've picked up this book, you are probably already starting on the journey into menopause. Menopause is an inevitable event in every woman's life. Some fear it; some welcome it. For some women, it is a relief; for others, the symptoms of menopause are life shattering. "The Change"—as it is so appropriately called—brings on a shift in many areas of a woman's life. It isn't just the end of the menses. It is a major transition into a new phase of life.

Our bodies are subject to rhythms and cycles. Once a woman starts menstruating in her teenage years, she can expect to experience a monthly cycle for somewhere between thirty-five and forty-five years. There can be pregnancies or changes that might cause the cycle to be irregular, but for most women, menses becomes a familiar friend. You set your calendar based on it. You know what to expect. You come to recognize the different signs as you shift from ovulation to menstrual flow.

Sometime between their late forties and mid-fifties, most women will start to notice changes in this cycle. By the time a woman reaches her midfifties, she will have entered into menopause. Some women have very few symptoms and hardy notice anything except that their cycle has stopped. Others have disabling symptoms and are in desperate need of help. Hot flashes, mood swings, sleep disturbances, changes in the vaginal tissues, loss of sexual desire, memory loss, weakening of bones: These symptoms can turn your life upside down.

The Conventional Approach

Conventional medicine has had one answer to help women during this time: hormone replacement therapy. It was estimated that in 1995, over 38 percent of postmenopausal women were using hormones to treat and prevent the symptoms of menopause. Some women have been taking hormones for more than twenty years on the recommendation of their physician.

In July 2002, the results of the Women's Health Initiative were published in the *Journal of the American Medical Association*. It sent a shock wave into the medical community and put fear and concern into every woman taking hormones for menopausal symptoms. The study was discontinued early because of the increase in invasive breast cancer, strokes, and blood clots noted among the women taking the combination formula of Premarin and Provera.

As a result of the study, many women stopped taking their hormones and are looking for alternatives to help get through these changes more gracefully. Many others decided not to start taking hormones in the first place.

It Takes More than Hormones

It takes more than just popping a few pills to maintain health during this second half of life. The earlier you start treating yourself well, the better these years will be. The way you live your life when it comes to your diet, exercise, and supplements can make a great difference in your overall health and well-being. The science of longevity is evolving, and we know that prevention of disease is more important than treating a disease once it exists.

A woman's life expectancy has radically increased over the last century. Now in the 21st century, a woman can expect to live a long, healthy life into her eighties, and maybe even nineties for our current generation. This means that many women will be living at least half or even more than half of their lives after menopause. Therefore, it is even more important for a woman to learn how to take care of herself. This book is a guide to help women navigate through the years of premenopause and menopause. You have the power to affect the way your body handles this change that is much more than taking a pill. What you eat, what supplements you take, and how you take care of yourself will all have a dramatic effect on your life. This book is a tool to guide you through this transition and into the second half of your life.

Many women in the early stages of premenopause and menopause are confused about what they can do to make the transition easier. The current conventional medical approach during these years is to use a low-dose birth control pill. For many women, this approach makes their symptoms worse, especially if they are the estrogen-dominant type. There are many other more natural alternatives to be found in the pages of this book.

Your unique medical history will shape your specific concerns. If many of your family members have had heart problems, then you will especially want to read the chapter on keeping your heart healthy. If you have had family members with Alzheimer's disease, perhaps keeping your mind sharp will be important. You might also find that in some cases, the recommendations are very similar since we know that antioxidants are very important for protecting both the heart and the brain.

The first chapter will help you find ways to ease menopause's early stages and even give you some suggestions to help you get the right tests done by your doctor. In the other chapters, you can read about specific symptoms and things that you can do to help keep your bones strong, protect your heart, or spice up your sex life.

Menopause is a time of great change in a woman's life. That is why it is referred to as the "Change of Life." Women do not only have physiological changes; powerful emotional and spiritual changes occur, as well, when a woman comes more into her strength and power.

As you pass through this amazing transition, learn how to turn it into a positive experience. We all want to live longer and healthier lives. This book is filled with tools to keep you healthy and vital. Menopause is an exciting and challenging time in a woman's life. Let this book guide you through it.

CHAPTER 1

PREMENOPAUSE AND MENOPAUSE: LIVING IN TRANSITION

Last week a friend came to me looking tired and concerned. "I don't know what's happening to me," she said. "I'm still having my period, but now I'm so hot, especially at night. I throw the covers off because I'm sweating, then I get freezing cold. I'm still having regular periods, though. Is this menopause? When does menopause start?"

For years before a woman goes into menopause, she may have problems as her hormones start to shift; this can be the beginning of menopause. We now use the term *perimenopause* for the changes in hormones that happen when a woman is still having periods.

The Cycle of Hormones

Luteal Phase
The second half of the menstrual cycle, from ovulation until the onset of the menstrual period.

The ovaries have a regular cycle as the hormones rise and fall. During the week of the menstrual cycle, hormone levels will be low. Then, at midcycle, sometime around day fourteen, estrogen will peak as an egg is released. This is called ovulation. During the second two weeks of the cycle, the ovary will produce estrogen and progesterone to prepare the uterus for the egg to implant. This time is called the luteal phase. In these approximately two weeks, the hormone levels will be at their highest. They will peak at between days twenty and twenty-four, and then fall over the next few days. When hormone levels fall, the menstrual period begins.

Depending upon the overall health of the woman and her body's ability to process these higher hormone levels, many fluctuations can occur. This is why so many women have different symptoms during this monthly ebb and flow. Hormones can have a dramatic effect on a woman's feeling of well-being, her moods, and her emotions. These hormone changes, when out of balance, can wreak havoc in a woman's life. She can feel totally out of control, wondering why she is doing things.

Because of the powerful effect that hormones have on our emotional life and stability, it is important for us to help educate each other and support each other as we move into this transition in life.

What Is Premenopause?

With menopause, a woman's ovaries stop releasing regular eggs every month. Before the ovaries stop altogether, the cycles will often be irregular. An egg might not be released every month, or the ovary may not produce enough hormones.

As a woman enters her forties, she may experience changes in her cycles. Some women will begin to have symptoms years before they go into full menopause. The symptoms during this time can include hot flashes, mood swings such as depression and irritability, sexual problems, and a worsening of PMS symptoms. There can even be patterns of irregular bleeding, which can range from longer cycles such as thirty-five to forty days or shorter cycles of twenty-one days or less.

This time is called premenopause. It refers to the time just before menopause when things start to change but there is still some type of a cycle. During premenopause, shifts will start to occur. Women may even skip a few months between periods, but then they start up again. When your period has stopped completely for six months, you can be considered officially in menopause. You may even have one or two more cycles, however, which can come even in the first or second year of menopause.

There are likely to be wide fluctuations in hormone levels during premenopause. Some women will have very high estrogen and progesterone; others will experience just the opposite, with very low hormonal levels.

The best way to tell where you are in this process is to have your hormones tested. If you are still having periods, I recommend getting two different tests. Most doctors will only check your FSH, follicle stimulating hormone, and maybe estradiol on the second or third day of bleeding. This is a good way to determine your fertility and also to see how close you are to menopause. FSH levels rise higher the closer you get to menopause as the pituitary attempts to stimulate the ovary to release more eggs. In premenopause, FSH will be above 25 ng/ml. Once the ovary has no more eggs to release, the levels of estrogen will fall and the FSH will soar above 50 ng/ml.

Follicle Stimulating Hormone (FSH)

A hormone secreted by the pituitary at midcycle to stimulate the release of an egg from the ovary.

For women in premenopause still having cycles but experiencing fluctuations in hormones, I often also check levels during the luteal phase, the second half of the cycle. The ideal time is between five days and one week before the menses is going to start. This is when the hormone levels are at their peak. Whether the hormone levels are high or low at this time can reveal a lot about why you may be having problems.

The Change Begins

With the maturing of the baby boom generation, attitudes toward women and "The Change" have dramatically changed. The largest population of women is entering menopause—and they want to talk about it! Now with the new research from the Women's Health Initiative and the Heart and Estrogen/Progestin Replacement Study (HERS Study), we can expect things to change even more.

We are the generation of the women's movement. Unlike many of our mothers, we are in the workplace expecting to be treated equally to men. We are able to talk openly about our symptoms. We won't "suffer in silence" the way our mothers did.

Many women are approaching this time in their life looking for alternatives to conventional hormone replacement therapy. Conventional hormones have been associated with side effects and complications. Many women don't want to take the risk. Although HRT may be beneficial for some, it is not for every woman.

Even if you decide to use HRT, other factors are important to maintain health and vitality. It takes a lot more than just a pill to make the years after menopause productive and exciting. This book can be your guide to keeping young and vital, even beyond menopause.

These are the recommended tests to have done to evaluate your hormone levels. If these tests show that you are having low or high levels, and you're experiencing symptoms during your cycle, hormonal or herbal support may be warranted.

Day 2–3 of cycle	Measure FSH and estradiol
Day 20–24 of a regular cycle	Measure estradiol and progesterone
Other hormones to test	Testosterone, DHEA-S, pregnenolone

CHAPTER 2

HORMONE REPLACEMENT THERAPY: YES OR NO?

Over the past twenty to thirty years, the medical community has been prescribing hormone replacement for women in menopause. Up until July 2002, HRT was considered the panacea for women to prevent heart disease, osteoporosis, and the symptoms of menopause. Estrogen therapy is helpful for many women and has been the treatment of choice for millions of women after menopause. There are also many women who have had their ovaries removed or who had an early menopause. Many of these women have been using estrogen for twenty to thirty years.

The transition into menopause has a wide range of effects for women. Some won't even notice that it is happening and are grateful to be relieved of their monthly flow. For others, however, there will be uncomfortable symptoms that will make their life torturous. It is clear that hormones are effective for relieving symptoms and helping with osteoporosis, but they will not protect the heart and may increase the risk of cancer in some women.

Osteoporosis
A condition of progressive bone loss that leads to spontaneous fractures.

The Latest Research on Hormones

When the results of the research study from the Women's Health Initiative indicated that women using estrogens might increase their risk of hormone-related cancers, it sent shock waves into the medical community. Thousands of women stopped taking their hormones upon the advice of their doctor—or just stopped all together without even talking with their doctor out of fear.

In the research study, women taking a combination of Premarin with Provera—a product called Prempro—had a higher rate of breast cancer. There were thirty-eight invasive breast cancer cases per ten thousand women, compared to the control group of thirty cases per ten thousand. Eight more cases represents a 26 percent increase in the rate of cancer. Because of this increase, the study was discontinued. Since then, the U.S. Food and Drug Administration has decided to put a warning label on any products containing estrogens, stating that they may increase the risk of cancer. The study with women who have had a hysterectomy who are using estrogen only—namely, Premarin—continues. It appears from this that it was the progestin in the study that increased the risk of cancer, not the estrogen.

The other important development in the study is that there was also a significant increase in the formation of blood clots, pulmonary embolism, and strokes. Estrogen, especially when taken in capsule form, can increase the production of factors that increase clotting in the blood by the liver. This has been known for years, since the development of the birth control pill. In the early research on birth control, the high doses of estrogen used in the pills were shown to cause an increase in clots that could lead to phlebitis in the legs and cause clots to enter the lungs or brain. This study confirmed that Prempro could also increase the risk of these problems, especially among those who are at risk for these blood clots.

Pulmonary Embolism
Blood clots that form in the legs or heart and travel to the lungs, blocking arteries and causing a lack of oxygen.

This particular research study used only Premarin and Prempro, a combination of Premarin and medroxyprogesterone. This product contains conjugated estrogens from the urine of pregnant mares.

These estrogens are metabolized differently in the liver than are the natural estrogens that the ovaries manufacture. They tend to be stronger and often have more side effects than the natural biologically identical hormones.

The progesterone product in Prempro—medroxy-progesterone—is a synthetic form and has more side effects than does natural micronized progesterone. Medroxyprogesterone can cause weight gain, headaches, bloating, depression, and breast tenderness. From a report from the Mayo Clinic, 80 percent of women reported feeling better on natural micronized progesterone compared to synthetic.

One of the major issues with the Women's Health Initiative and its interpretation is this: Currently, there is no evidence that other forms of estrogen and progesterone—especially when used in the biologically identical forms—increase the risks of breast cancer, stroke, or blood clots at the same rate. Nonetheless, there are concerns about estrogen and its potential cancer risk.

The other issue is the exposure to environmental hormones and chemicals called xenoestrogens. There is a concern that this exposure, when added to hormone replacement—or even to the estrogens consumed through a woman's life, such as by taking birth control pills for many years—could be the reason we are seeing such an increase in breast cancer.

Xenoestrogens
Chemicals that are synthetically produced and have an estrogen-like effect on the cells.

Overall, whether you should take estrogen or not, and in what form, will need to be an individual decision based upon your unique situation. If you have a family history of breast cancer, it might be wise to look at options besides using estrogen. Even if you don't have such a family history, there may still be concerns, since many women currently being diagnosed with breast cancer have not had breast cancer in their family. The overall lifetime risk of breast cancer is one in eight to ten. If you have a family history

BRCA 1 and 2 Gene
Genes that are involved in cell growth but that, when are present in your DNA and mutated, will increase your risk of breast cancer.

and carry the BRCA 1 or 2 gene, that risk increases to a 50 to 85 percent chance of developing breast cancer. Read more about this in Chapter 9.

Is Estrogen the Only Way?

The medical treatment of menopause has truly focused only on estrogen as the one hormone that can fix the symptoms. Estrogen helps with sleep disturbance, hot flashes, mood swings, vaginal dryness, memory problems, and osteoporosis. Though all of these things are true, there may be ways to help these symptoms and improve the quality of life for women after menopause that don't involve using estrogen. There are also other hormones that can be combined with estrogen in smaller doses.

If we examine the way our bodies make and use other hormones, it is evident that there are many steps before estrogen is produced. Several other hormones, such as progesterone, pregnenolone, dihydro-epiandrosterone (DHEA), and testosterone, are also produced by the ovaries and in the adrenal glands. Levels of these hormones can be measured in the blood; you can see how much of these you are still making. If your levels are low, these hormones can be taken as supplements. DHEA, pregnenolone, and lower dosages of progesterone are available over the counter and can be found in capsules, sublingual drops, or creams. The resource section in the back of this book lists sources of quality products.

In theory, after menopause, hormone production is supposed to be taken over by the adrenal glands. The adrenal glands produce DHEA, testosterone, and pregnenolone, and may even produce small amounts of estrogen and progesterone. It is also believed that progesterone, testosterone, and DHEA will turn into estrogen as they are metabolized. Estrogen is produced in small amounts in fat cells, as well.

Before taking any estrogen product, make sure to have your estradiol level measured by your doctor. Checking FSH levels alone isn't enough to tell you if you need to take estrogen.

Many women are concerned about taking estrogen because of the latest research, but there are some who have such severe symptoms that small dosages of estrogen can make a huge difference in their lives and sense of well-being. Debilitating hot flashes, severe depression and irritability, osteoporosis, or vaginal dryness with sexual problems will be helped with estrogen replacement.

If you need to take estrogen, use the lowest possible dosage and look at combining it with other hormones such as progesterone, testosterone, DHEA, or pregnenolone. Each of these has a separate effect, and you might have a better overall result if you combine these natural hormones instead of using estrogen alone. There are also different forms of estrogen available. Two other natural forms are used for hormone replacement: estriol and estrone. Estradiol can be found in combinations with estriol (called Bi-est), or with estriol and estrone (Tri-est). Read more about these below.

Estradiol is a natural form of estrogen that is produced in the body. It is available in patch form, and also as a tablet. A compounding pharmacy can make up estradiol for you in the form of a smaller-dosage capsule, a cream, or sublingual drops. Creams, drops, and patches all bypass the liver for those women who have trouble digesting or don't absorb well. If you are going to take estradiol, try to use the lowest possible dosage that still helps control your symptoms. A simple blood test can tell you if you are getting too much.

Estriol: The Forgotten Estrogen?

Estriol is a weaker form of estrogen produced by the ovaries. It was extensively studied in the 1960s and has been researched in Asia and Europe as beneficial for the symptoms of menopause. Estriol use is being revived in the United States as an alternative to the other forms of estrogen available.

Estriol is the predominant form of estrogen produced during pregnancy. It is found in high concentrations in the amniotic fluid that bathes the fetus. Estriol is a weaker estrogen converted from estrone and androstenedione. It competes with the same receptor sites as estradiol.

In a landmark article published in 1966 in the *Journal of the American Medical Association*, Dr. Henry Lemon described estriol as a nontoxic physiologic antagonist for ovarian estrogens. He found that estriol provided benefits for postmenopausal women, as it appeared to protect the uterus and breast. Because of the unique effect of estriol on the cells, it is believed to offer less of a risk for causing cancer of the uterine lining and breast.

Dr. Lemon used estriol on animals treated with cancer-causing chemicals and radiation. Estriol caused a more mature breast cancer cell to form, and as a result there was a reduction in the development of tumors in these animals. Although there are few human studies on the cancer-preventing effects of estriol, German gynecologist Christian Lauritzen, M.D., treated 940 women with 2 mg of estriol for five years. The women experienced relief from menopausal symptoms. Only two cases of breast cancer occurred when statistically three were expected, and no cases of endometrial cancer occurred when three were expected. Certainly this is a smaller study than the Women's Health Initiative, but it is very encouraging.

Dr. Lemon even hypothesized that estriol may have a protective effect against breast cancer. In his research, he found that women who produce less estriol compared to estradiol and estrone have an increased risk of developing breast cancer. In fact, in 1975 he used estriol to treat twenty-eight women with breast cancer and reported that 37 percent went into remission. More studies on the use of estriol and cancer have not been published, but with many women using estriol, there may soon be more information available on its cancer-protective effects. Estriol is still an estrogen, and how it is metabolized by the liver may be important in determining its anti-cancer effects.

Estriol has been used successfully to reverse the vaginal dryness from menopause without thickening the uterine lining. Several studies on using estriol to treat hot flashes and vaginal dryness have shown results similar to estradiol's.

Whether estriol (like estradiol) will protect against osteoporosis is not clear. In early studies done in Japan, estriol did not appear to be effective in improving bone density. This was discouraging, but another study from Italy using vaginal estriol showed that it was somewhat effective. A study from Taiwan using estriol succinate did not produce positive results on bone density.

If you have osteoporosis or are concerned about losing bone mass and want to use estriol, monitor your bone density, and have a urine test for N-telopeptide done periodically. This test uses the second morning urine to tell you if you are continuing to lose bone. Remember to incorporate the other things to help your bone density mentioned in Chapter 7.

N-telopeptide
A protein released with the breakdown of bone. Elevated levels in the urine indicate excessive bone loss.

Some women might experience fewer side effects with estriol and could try using this form of estrogen instead of some of the stronger alternatives. Like other estrogens, Estriol can cause breast tenderness, bloating, and weight gain. The dosage of estriol is usually higher than estradiol. Estriol can be taken orally or used in a topical cream. Dosages of 1–5 mg daily have been effective. For vaginal atrophy, 0.5 mg per gram of cream can be inserted several times per week. Estriol is a wonderful alternative to estradiol or other synthetic estrogens.

Tri-Est and Bi-Est

Several years ago, a combination of natural, biologically identical hormones was determined to be the ideal mixture of hormones for a woman. It consisted of 80 percent concentration of estriol with 10 percent concentration of estradiol and estrone. This has been the most widely used compounded prescription for women desiring a natural hormone formula. The most common dosage is 1.25–2.5 mg once or twice a day. It is usually combined with the appropriate dosage of progesterone, testosterone, and DHEA to make a great formula for women in menopause.

Those women who have not been helped sufficiently with this formula and are still experiencing vaginal dryness, hot flashes, or mood swings might try using a different formula of just estriol and estradiol called Bi-est. This formula contains 80 percent estriol and 20 percent estradiol. Since many women manufacture excess amounts of estrone after menopause, I have chosen to prescribe the Bi-est formula for most women, avoiding additional estrone.

Levels of estradiol, estrone, and estriol can be measured to determine the metabolism of these estrogens. The way the body clears these estrogens becomes essential. It may not necessarily be just the hormones themselves but what the body does with them that makes the difference in the risk of cancer. Read more about this in Chapter 9.

All about Testosterone

Anabolic Steroid
A hormone with a cholesterol structure that is responsible for building proteins and muscle.

We think of testosterone as a male hormone, but in fact it is a very important hormone for women, as well. Testosterone is an anabolic steroid hormone. It is responsible for libido, sexual response, and orgasm. Levels of testosterone will often fall in premenopause and menopause.

Symptoms of low testosterone include depression, apathy, difficulty with concentration, fatigue, low libido, and difficulty with orgasm.

Testosterone increases muscle mass and strength.

It also reduces cholesterol, triglycerides, and blood sugar. Because testosterone will increase muscle mass and strength, it will also affect metabolism. A condition called Syndrome X that has become epidemic in our society features obesity, high blood pressure, and high blood sugar. This condition has been linked to low testosterone. When testosterone levels are higher, there will be lower insulin resistance and body fat with an improvement in overall health.

Insulin Resistance
An elevated level of insulin with an increase in insulin receptors such that the cells do not respond to the insulin as they should.

Another myth about testosterone is that it is dangerous for the heart. The truth is that testosterone appears to help circulation and actually causes the arteries to dilate. One study on men with angina found that those treated with testosterone had fewer episodes of chest pain. In fact, most men develop heart disease as they become older and their testosterone levels fall.

Angina
A medical condition in which the blood vessels providing oxygen and nutrients to the heart spasm and cause chest pain.

Replacement of testosterone can be beneficial for most women after menopause and even during premenopause. There are several ways you can take testosterone. It is available in creams, capsules, or sublingual drops. Most doctors agree that taking testosterone in either cream or sublingual drop form is probably best so that more of it will get into the bloodstream and bypass the liver.

There can be many benefits to using testosterone as a part of hormone replacement therapy, or even using small amounts of it instead of estrogen. Some women have reported doing very well using only progesterone and testosterone. Among some women, testosterone will be converted into small amounts of estrogen, so they should watch out for estrogen's side effects such as breast tenderness, bloating, weight gain, or water retention.

There is also another form of testosterone that has become more popular for women who have had breast cancer: Methyltestosterone can be compounded into creams, drops, or lozenges. Because of its unique biochemical structure, this form of testosterone will not be converted into estrogen and is considered safer for women who have had estrogen-receptor-positive cancers. For women with breast cancer, testosterone or methyltestosterone can be helpful in alleviating hot flashes and vaginal dryness, and will even help maintain bone mass. Methyltestosterone is also available in Estratest, a combination with conjugated estrogens.

It is always best to start with low dosages of testosterone and watch for side effects. I usually recommend using 0.5–1 mg daily to start. Rarely are dosages higher than 10 mg daily prescribed for women.

Testosterone can cause masculinizing side effects such as acne, increased facial hair, hair loss, irritability, or enlargement of the clitoris. In high dosages, it can cause the voice to become deeper. Most of the time, these side effects are reversible when caught early.

Many women feel great using testosterone, and the hormone is critical in reviving the waning libido and sexual response that can come with menopause. Besides the sexual benefits, testosterone can lift your mood and restore your interest and excitement in life.

DHEA: The Hormone for Vitality

DHEA is produced primarily in the adrenal glands. As the years have passed, we have found out more about this amazing hormone. Research shows that DHEA levels fall with aging and illness, especially autoimmune disease. When there is prolonged stress, the adrenal glands will become fatigued and will not be able to maintain production of DHEA.

Several studies have looked at replacing DHEA in people with lower-than-normal blood levels. The results were impressive. Patients reported better sleep, better energy, and improved function of the immune system. In a double-blind crossover study reported in *Annals of New York Academy of Science* in 1995, thirty subjects aged forty through seventy used 50 mg daily for three months. Sixty-seven percent of the men and 84 percent of the women reported improved physical and psychological well-being. During the study, no side effects were reported. In other research, patients with lupus, rheumatoid arthritis, autoimmune hemolytic anemia, and multiple sclerosis report reduced immune complex formation, increased stamina, and improved well-being with replacement to normal physiological levels.

DHEA is available over the counter or by prescription from a compounding pharmacy. It is best to start with small dosages, such as 5–10 mg daily. Most over-the-counter preparations are available in 25 mg. A few are available at this lower dosage, or you may need to order it from the compounding pharmacy. Since DHEA can be converted into either estrogen or testosterone, there are several things to watch if you are going to take it as a supplement.

First, always begin by having your doctor check DHEA-S levels to see if yours are low. Levels will fall as you get older, are under stress, or become ill. Low levels are associated with fatigue, lowered immune function, poor sleep, and a loss of the sense of well-being.

Side effects of DHEA could be related to excess testosterone or excess estrogen. Women can develop acne, increased facial hair, or even hair loss when they start taking supplemental DHEA. Symptoms associated with too much estrogen—breast tenderness, bloating, or weight gain—could occur. Ovarian cysts, weight gain, and acne are symptoms of an overproduction of DHEA in women.

On the positive side, many people report feeling better when their level of DHEA returns to normal. DHEA supplementation is a good alternative to the use of estrogen replacement. Currently, legislation is pending that might make DHEA supplements illegal.

Up until now, they have been available over the counter.

High Estrogen: Too Much of a Good Thing

In the early stages of menopause and pre-menopause, most women will continue to make some estrogen. In some cases, estrogen levels can become so high that it can be very uncomfortable. Symptoms of excess estrogen can include bloating, water retention, breast tenderness, fibrocystic breasts, carbohydrate carvings, ovarian cysts, irregular bleeding, uterine fibroids, irritability, and depression. During premenopause, estrogen levels can become 200–300 ng/dl higher than normal. This can further create difficulties.

Often, the ovaries are not producing an egg each month, so there isn't enough progesterone produced to balance the estrogen. Many women complain of the symptoms of estrogen excess during this time. In the last ten years, it has become more common for doctors to prescribe low-dose birth control pills for women experiencing premenopausal symptoms. The pill prevents some of the problems associated with irregular bleeding. Unfortunately, if there is excess estrogen and low progesterone, the pill can make some symptoms worse.

One approach for women who are having this problem is to measure levels of estrogen and progesterone about three weeks after the first day of the menstrual cycle. When estrogen is high and progesterone is low, there are several things to do.

First, you can use herbs to lower estrogen levels. Since estrogen is cleared by the liver, using herbs that help support liver function will help the body clear excess estrogen. Formulas that help the liver break down fats are beneficial. These usually include several herbs that help the liver, such as dandelion, beet root, and milk thistle. Two other supplements commonly used for high estrogen are calcium d-glucarate and indole 3-carbinol or di-indole-methane. There is more information on these in Chapter 9.

To raise progesterone levels, use one of the over-the-counter creams; if your levels are very low, you might need to have your doctor order a prescription for progesterone. Herbs such as vitex can help raise progesterone levels. Since progesterone requires B_6 and magnesium, adding these to your supplement regimen can also help counter waning levels.

When trying to decide whether or not to use hormone replacement, it is important to consider your family history, your medical history, and overall symptoms. If there are other alternatives to try, you might see if some of the other hormones will suffice, or try lower dosages. If you are using prescription hormones, use the lowest possible dosage of estrogen that you need to control your symptoms.

CHAPTER 3

HERBAL ALTERNATIVES

Many women have chosen not to take hormones in natural or synthetic form and have taken the herbal route. Herbal medicine has been used for centuries and has been helpful to women from cultures around the world. The Indian, Asian, and Native American cultures all have a tradition of using herbs to help women as they grow into the wise woman stage of their lives. Women in these cultures were honored for their knowledge and experience. Now with women living to an average age of seventy-nine, some are living more than half their lives after menopause. We need ways to stay healthy, and herbal medicines may be a solution.

Plant-based medicine has been studied for years, and the composition of many herbs is now well known. Research in herbal medicine also continues all over the world: We now know more about herbs than ever before. Plants that are used as medicines are rich in vitamins, minerals, and substances called alkaloids that are specific to each plant. Many herbs contain substances that thin the blood or would be contraindicated if you are taking prescription medicines. Before taking any herbal medication, make sure you review any potential side effects with your doctor.

Alkaloids
Nitrogen-containing substances found in plants that are specific to each individual plant species.

Herbal combinations work best, but there are some herbs that are effective even alone. Look for herbs that are standardized to a certain concentration of active ingredient. Herbal remedies come as capsules or liquid tinctures, or can be made into teas. They are usually most effective when taken several times daily.

Although herbal remedies are very popular and effective in some cases to control hot flashes and vaginal dryness, there is no indication that they will help maintain bone mass. If you are at risk for osteoporosis and using herbal remedies, have your bone density tested periodically, and have the urine test done that measures N-telopeptide (see Chapter 7). Make sure you are taking extra nutrients to maintain your bones.

Black Cohosh

Black cohosh (*Cimicifuga racemosa*) is an herb that Native Americans used for many things, including various female problems. It has estrogen-like activity, but the exact mechanism is unknown. It is an anti-inflammatory and actually contains small amounts of natural salicylic acid, the active ingredient in aspirin. It is useful for menstrual cramps, as well as many symptoms of menopause. Black cohosh is also used for headaches, muscle cramps, and arthritis.

The most commonly used form of black cohosh for menopause is Remifemin. This product, from Enzymatic Therapy, is a standardized extract containing 20 mg of black cohosh with 1 mg of triterpene glycosides. In a clinical study of 152 patients treated with 20–40 mg daily for twelve weeks, 80 percent reported improvement of menopausal symptoms. There was no increase in the growth of estrogen-sensitive cancer cells when they were exposed to black cohosh extract.

It still is not known whether black cohosh is safe for women who have been treated for breast cancer, but many oncologists are permitting their patients to try it for their symptoms. Side effects of black cohosh include nausea, vomiting, dizziness, and nervous system and visual disturbances.

Red Clover

Another herb rich in phytoestrogens is red clover (*Trifolium pratense*). It is rich in isoflavones that have estrogenic activity. The most common product available over the counter is Promensil, a standardized extract with 80 mg of red clover isoflavones. There is currently no research data on long-term use of red clover.

Red clover contains substances that could slow down the clotting of blood, so caution should be used if you are taking other medications to thin the blood, such as Coumadin. It also can slow down the metabolism of certain drugs that use the cytochrome p450 enzymes. Check with your doctor or pharmacist if there might be a problem.

Cytochrome p450 enzymes
Enzymes in the liver that are responsible for the detoxification of drugs and chemicals.

Siberian Ginseng

Siberian ginseng is from a different species than the other ginsengs and is used slightly differently. It is an excellent tonic for weakening adrenal glands. It can help provide energy and stamina but without being overstimulating. It is safe for long-term use and can even be used by children with recurrent infections to improve the immune system.

Adaptogen
An herbal medicine that increases the resistance and creates a balance to lower abnormally high levels and raise abnormally low levels.

Siberian ginseng is especially helpful for women during periods of stress and in menopause. It is considered an adaptogen and has antiviral activity. Since it can support adrenal function, it can improve adrenal hormone function. It may have some estrogen-like effects, although that is not its primary action.

Siberian ginseng can be taken as a powder with 0.3 percent eleutheroside at 400 mg per day or a liquid tincture between $\frac{1}{2}$ and 3 teaspoons three times daily. Although it is not as stimulating as the other ginsengs, it can exacerbate heart palpitations, anxiety, or other heart problems. Use it cautiously if you have any of these symptoms. In general, it is excellent to combine with other herbs such as licorice, rhodiola, or American ginseng.

American Ginseng

American ginseng root (*Panax ginseng*) is a different species of ginseng from the Korean or Chinese root. Native to the northern United States, this form of ginseng is better suited for women than the others. American ginseng is used as a tonic to improve resistance to stress and immune function. It has estrogenic action and so can be beneficial for women in menopause. Research studies show that American ginseng may decrease the growth of breast cancer cells, but because of its estrogenic activity it should be used with caution in women with hormone-sensitive cancers.

American ginseng does not have the same side effects as the other, stronger species. It can still be stimulating—it should be used cautiously in the presence of heart conditions—and may interact with some medications. It can be used in combination with other herbs such as Siberian ginseng, dong quai, vitex, or licorice. The usual dosage is 250–500 mg two times daily.

Dong Quai

Dong quai is a root found in the Chinese herbal medicine tradition and known for its blood-building qualities. It is recommended for anemia and for women who tend to be cold and tired, especially around their menses. It improves circulation and contains iron and vitamin B_{12}. It is a tonic often used after childbirth to help build blood.

Women experiencing excess bleeding should not use dong quai except in small quantities as part of a balanced formula. It does not contain phytoestrogens, but the components in the root can help raise estrogen levels during premenopause and menopause. The usual dose of dong quai is 3–4 grams daily when taken alone. Smaller doses would be used if taken in a combination.

Deer Antler

Deer antler is a tonic that has been part of the Chinese tradition for more than three thousand years. Rich in amino acids, vitamins, and minerals, it is known for its rejuvenative qualities. It has been known to increase the production of hormones and even contains some estrogen. It also contains growth factors that may increase the level of growth hormone. Deer antler velvet enriches the blood by stimulating white and red blood cell production.

The extract from the tips of the antlers is used. Deer shed their antlers each year, and when the new growth returns, the tips are harvested. The deer are not harmed in the process. Many research studies on using deer antler extract have been performed, most of them focusing on the components of this extract that help increase growth hormone production and improve athletic performance. It has been useful in increasing testosterone levels in men. A dosage of 500 mg is recommended.

Licorice

Licorice root has a long tradition in Chinese and traditional Western herbology. It has many uses, including aiding digestion and the secretion of bile. It is antiviral, anti-inflammatory, and helps support the adrenal glands. Licorice contains specific isoflavones that are estrogenic. Too much licorice can lower potassium levels or raise blood pressure.

Licorice makes a very sweet tea; it can also be taken in capsules of 500 mg two to three times daily, or as a liquid tincture. Because of its potential side effects, it's best to use licorice in smaller amounts with other synergistic herbs such as dong quai, black cohosh, or ginseng.

Maca Root

Maca root (*Lepidium meyenii*) is thought of as the vitality secret of the Incas. It is a tuber growing in high mountains of Peru. Maca is very rich in nutrients including proteins, calcium, magnesium, phosphorus, iodine, thiamin, riboflavin, and vitamin C. It also contains specific alkaloids and polysaccharides. In animal studies, those animals given maca root showed improved fertility. Research shows that maca supports the endocrine system by supporting the hypothalamus and pituitary to enhance hormone synthesis.

Polysaccharide
Long chains of sugars linked together that have specific chemical actions.

Unlike many other herbs used for menopause, it does not appear that maca contains phytoestrogens; instead, it helps the adrenals and ovaries increase their hormone production. Maca can be used to relieve vaginal dryness, ease hot flashes, and improve libido. It can be taken as powder mixed in juice or capsules. The usual dosage is 500 mg–2 grams daily.

Vitex

Vitex agnus-castus is an aromatic tree that grows in the Mediterranean. It was once used by monks to lower their libido. The berries contain the active ingredients viticine and casticin.

Vitex has been used to raise progesterone levels, and in research studies was found to improve estrogen and progesterone levels in women having irregular periods. It is especially useful for women in premenopause who have low progesterone levels. The dosage is 120–500 mg daily in capsules or liquid tincture.

Conclusion

Herbal combinations have been around for thousands of years. Cultures from around the world feature traditions of using herbal medicines to help women from pregnancy into menopause. Given today's revived interest in herbal medicine and the need for alternatives to conventional HRT, herbs may well be the answer for millions of women looking for symptom relief with health benefits. We continue to learn more about the amazing substances in herbal medicines, these powerful gifts from Mother Nature.

CHAPTER 4

IS IT HOT IN HERE OR IS IT ME? CONTROLLING HOT FLASHES

Hot flashes—those waves of heat that rise from your toes to your head, making you turn completely red and break out into a sweat—are extremely uncomfortable. They're even worse when they occur in the night and interfere with sleep. Not all women have hot flashes during menopause, but many have such debilitating episodes that their lives become miserable.

To date, there is no exact knowledge on what causes hot flashes. The phenomenon is believed to occur when the temperature center in the hypothalamus loses its regulation. The body becomes excessively hot and produces sweat to cool off. Then you get cold and chills. These changes in temperature can happen up to twenty times in one hour.

Although the main reason for hot flashes has been thought to be lower estrogen levels, low progesterone and even high estrogen levels can also cause them. Some women get hot flashes even while they are still having regular periods. In premenopause, hot flashes will most commonly occur just before or during the flow. This is because of the lower level of hormones during this time. Hormone replacement therapy is one of the most effective treatments to alleviate hot flashes. Both estradiol and estriol have been found to be helpful in reducing hot flashes. But if you are a woman who has chosen not to use estrogen, don't despair. There are a number of other alternatives.

The other hormones mentioned in Chapter 2 can

also help with hot flashes. Natural progesterone in creams or capsules has been shown to reduce hot flashes. Several companies produce a high-quality cream containing progesterone. Most of the over-the-counter creams contain 25–30 mg of progesterone per $\frac{1}{4}$ teaspoon. The cream is applied twice daily. Creams with a higher concentration of progesterone are available from compounding pharmacies by prescription. Progesterone in capsules or sublingual drops can also help control hot flashes.

Progesterone is available by prescription as Promethium in 100 and 200 mg capsules. It is made in peanut oil so it cannot be used by anyone with a peanut allergy. It can also be formulated in other oils and at the desired dosage by a compounding pharmacy.

Testosterone helps reduce hot flashes, as well, and can be taken in small doses to avoid side effects. DHEA supplements may also help, since they will produce estrogen and testosterone. For some women, though, even the lowest dosage can cause side effects, so be aware of what they are (see Chapter 2).

Many of the herbs mentioned in the third chapter will help relieve hot flashes, especially when combined with progesterone. Certain vitamins are also beneficial, including vitamin E, pantothenic acid, and essential fatty acids.

There are a number of other things you can do to ward off those hot flashes. First, plan what you are wearing. Don't wear a wool turtleneck sweater if you will be in a warm room. Wear layers—jackets and sweaters that can be taken off. Put on lightweight tops or camisoles underneath blouses that you can remove when the heat comes.

Avoid excessively hot drinks and spicy foods—or if you do indulge, be ready to peel off some of those layers. Alcohol will also bring on flashes. Victoria's Secret makes a line of pajamas that feature a camisole with a jacket. These pajamas are great for those middle-of-the-night heat waves.

For most women, hot flashes are a temporary phenomenon that ease as the body adjusts to lower levels of hormones in the blood. Still, some women have hot flashes that persist for years. The less stress you have and the better you can take care of yourself, the more they should lessen over time.

CONTROLLING HOT FLASHES: SUPPLEMENT DOSAGE	
Vitamin E	400–1,200 IU daily
Pantothenic acid	500 mg daily
Essential fatty acids	300–400 mg GLA daily
Siberian ginseng	500 mg daily
Licorice root	500 mg 2 times daily
Maca	500 mg–2 grams daily
Natural progesterone	25–100 mg daily

CHAPTER 5

A HEALTHY DIET FOR LIFE

You are what you eat: This slogan from the 1970s has certainly proven to be true. Many research studies have supported the idea that people whose diets center on whole foods rich in nutrients enjoy better health. A recent study reported in the June 2002 *Journal of the American Medical Association* showed that a diet high in antioxidant foods can reduce your risk of Alzheimer's disease. As it turns out, the best diet is one high in fresh foods with an abundance of fruits and vegetables.

Make a Healthy Diet Your Habit

The healthiest diet for a healthy life is high in fruits and vegetables, whole grains, and lean meats. Vegetables and fruits are chock-full of vitamins and minerals that are antioxidants. The naturally occurring chemicals that give fruits and vegetables their wonderful bright red, orange, and yellow colors are flavonoids, which have powerful antioxidant activity. Antioxidants protect the cells and keep them vital. The fiber in fruits and vegetables helps the colon function better. This fiber helps keep the microorganisms in the colon alive, as well as absorbing excess chemicals that the body needs to clear.

Flavonoids *Chemical compounds found in plants that have specific effects and antioxidant activity, as well as bright color.*

Specific vegetables that are part of the cruciferous vegetable family have substances that help reduce the risk of cancer. The vegetables in this family are broccoli, Brussels sprouts, cabbage, and cauliflower. They contain a substance called indole 3-carbinol (I 3 C), which helps in the conversion of estrogen into forms less likely to cause cancer.

Whole grains are a rich source of B vitamins and minerals. They are found in the outer shell of grains—which also is rich in fiber. These grains are chock-full of nutrition to help with energy, as well as supporting nerve function. They also contain essential fatty acids. Whole-grain products are far and away more nutritious than their refined counterparts. Try switching to whole-grain breads and cereals instead of the highly refined white flours in your diet.

Soy: Yes or No?

Soy has benefits for some—but it's not for everyone. Many people use soy as a major source of protein in their diet. Soy has some limitations, however, so be aware that you might be eating too much of it. It can be very difficult to digest, for example; if you experience bloating after eating soy, you are probably not digesting it well and should avoid it.

Soy products contain phytoestrogens. This group of chemicals, called isoflavones, have an estrogen-like chemical structure. The action of these chemicals is like that of a weak estrogen. Although not as strong as regular estrogen, phytoestrogens can be taken in excess and still cause too much estrogen in the body. Breast tenderness, bloating, and excess bleeding are all signs that you are eating too much soy. Men can experience breast enlargement, sexual problems, and prostate enlargement.

There are several other problems with soy. For one, it contains very low amounts of methionine—one of the key amino acids that the liver requires to make glutathione, that organ's primary antioxidant. When there is too much soy in the diet and it is not well digested, health problems can occur that won't necessarily be linked to this dietary habit.

On the positive side, soy contains genistein, which helps the immune system. As a source of nutrition, it may be good for some and not for others. Using soy as your main source of protein may not be as beneficial as eating a broader range of proteins.

The Good Fats

Not all fat is bad. In fact, certain fats are needed for our health and well-being. Known as essential fatty acids, they are found in vegetables, nuts, seeds, and (especially) fish.

These oils are crucial to the production of a group of chemicals in the body called prostaglandins. There are different types of prostaglandins in the body. Some cause inflammation and pain, and others reduce it. Omega-6 and omega-3 fatty acids produce the prostaglandins that reduce pain and inflammation.

Prostaglandins
A class of active substances with a specific carbon chemical structure present in many tissues that have various physiologic actions.

Flax seeds contain the omega-6 fatty acid linoleic acid. Evening primrose, black currant, and borage seed oil also contain gamma-linoleic acid or GLA. Some people—especially diabetics—don't have the ability to convert the omega-6 oils found in flax into the GLA needed by the body. For these people, it is better to take supplements of about 300 mg of GLA.

Fish oils are a rich source of essential fatty acids. These are important for reducing inflammation and pain in the muscles and joints. Fish is also a healthy source of protein, and its oils have a specific effect on platelets: They help lessen the ability of platelets to stick together. This not only helps with circulation, but also reduces damage to the heart.

Incorporating foods that are rich in these oils in your diet will provide you with many health benefits. Not only do they help with breast tenderness, but they will also prevent the pain from arthritis, reduce heart disease, and help the brain function better.

Although dairy products may be healthy for some, they contain saturated fat. These fats, besides increasing your risk of heart disease, also increase the inflammatory prostaglandins and therefore can cause arthritis and inflammation throughout the body, including the breasts. If you have tender breasts, cut down on dairy products in your diet. If you are using dairy, use only organic products from animals that are hormone-free.

Mineral-Rich Foods

Many of the foods found in the typical American diet are lacking in minerals. It is important to pay attention to adding mineral-rich foods to your diet. Unless vegetables are organically grown, they will not be as rich in their mineral content. In addition, the soil where vegetables are grown must be enriched with minerals, or they won't supply you with the minerals you need.

Given the infusion of refined foods and fast foods in the American diet, more people are mineral deficient these days than ever before. Minerals are important for everything from energy production to healthy bones, muscles, and joints, as well as healthy brain and liver function. Without minerals, it is impossible to sustain good health. Yet it can be difficult to detect deficiencies in a routine blood test.

Another reason to consume more minerals is loss due to both exercise and consumption of caffeine. When you exercise and sweat, minerals are lost and need to be replaced. And of course, we are a nation of coffee drinkers. Coffeehouses are sprouting up in every neighborhood, especially in large cities; coffee has become the new social drink. Between large amounts of caffeine in coffee and the caffeine added to sodas, the average consumption of caffeine-containing beverages in America is overwhelming.

One of the big problems with caffeine is that it causes excess minerals and vitamins to be lost in the urine. Unless you are taking additional supplements and eating a healthy diet, daily caffeine can lead to mineral and vitamin deficiencies that may lead to serious health problems.

Incorporating whole foods in your diet helps

maintain the supply of minerals that your body needs. Refined grains and sugars have had their minerals removed, whereas whole foods are rich in nutrients. The outer coating of whole grains contains magnesium and other minerals. Use whole-grain flour or eat whole grains instead of the refined version whenever possible.

Foods that are high in magnesium are also important to include in your diet. Magnesium is found in the center of chlorophyll and is responsible for its green color. Leafy green vegetables are rich in magnesium, as are beans and lentils. Nuts and seeds are another good source of minerals.

A Diet for a Long, Healthy Life

No matter what type of health problem you may have, the dietary recommendations across the board are the same: Eating at least five servings daily of fruits and vegetables is the goal. Keep processed foods and fast foods to a minimum. It's just common sense. Use whole grains instead of refined flours. White sugar is empty calories and robs your cells of vital nutrients, so the less you have in your diet, the better.

Hormone-free meats are more widely available and are preferred. Fresh fish provide EPA and DHA—two omega-3 polyunsaturated essential fatty acids. Avoid the deep-ocean fish that may be contaminated with mercury, such as tuna and swordfish. The smaller the fish, the less likely they are to have accumulated toxic metals in their tissues.

Taking additional supplements of some nutrients may be necessary even with the best diet. Depending upon your individual genetic and medical history, you may need to take extra vitamins. We know that folic acid and vitamin B_{12} are helpful for the heart and nervous system and may even help prevent cancer. For women of childbearing age, folic acid supplements can prevent neural tube defects and prevent cervical cancer. As we research this field, we find more and more benefits from taking vitamin supplements.

For example, it is difficult to get enough calcium and magnesium in your daily food intake to keep your bones strong and prevent osteoporosis. An antioxidant supplement may help your cells avoid damage from free radicals. We know that this helps prevent Alzheimer's disease and cancer. It's even helpful for beautiful skin. This is an ever-changing and evolving field as we learn more and more about the role of nutrition and diet in our health. Start with a healthy diet as the basis for your vitality and well-being.

CHAPTER 6

HEALTHY BREASTS

One of the biggest concerns of women as they age is the risk of developing breast cancer. The rate of this cancer has increased in the last forty years. In 1960, one in every twenty women was diagnosed with breast cancer. Today, that has increased to one in every eight to ten women. Breast cancer remains the leading cause of death in women between the ages of thirty-five and fifty-four. The good news is that because of early diagnosis, more women are surviving breast cancer.

Certainly, the recent study revealing an increase in invasive breast cancer among women taking Prempro has many women concerned. They have stopped taking their hormones. Besides just cancer, many women develop cysts or fibrous areas in the breast that are benign. Fibrocystic breasts are very common in premenopausal women. There are many ways you can reduce your overall risk of cancer or fibrocystic breasts.

Estrogen definitely causes the breast tissue to be stimulated. When estrogen levels are high, the breasts will often become tender and form cysts. If you are having symptoms of fibrocystic breasts and are taking hormones, you can try going off estrogen all together, or reducing your dosage. One of my menopausal patients on HRT developed benign lumps in her breast, for example. When she went off her estrogen but stayed on her progesterone and added maca root, the cysts went away and she didn't suffer from severe menopausal symptoms.

The Role of Progesterone and the Breasts

Progesterone is one of the hormones that can reduce breast tenderness and reduce the formation of cysts. In premenopause, estrogen levels often become high while the progesterone levels are low. This is when taking supplements that help clear the estrogen and adding progesterone can help reduce pain, swelling, and cyst formation in the breasts.

Because progesterone can be converted into estrogen, it can cause the breasts to become tender in some women. Among women who are estrogen dominant, their metabolic pathways may send progesterone immediately into the production of more estrogen. These women surely need the progesterone, but must start slowly. If you develop sore breasts when you start taking progesterone, just start with a smaller dosage. Increase the dosage slowly to see how much your system will need.

A dose of 25 mg daily is a good place to start. Some women need as much as 100–400 mg daily. If you are at risk for high estrogen, you can keep your estrogen levels from becoming too high.

Lower Your Estrogen Levels

One of the major risk factors in breast problems is not only high estrogen but also the types of estrogen present in the body. Whether you are producing estrogen from the ovaries or taking estrogen, the liver needs to break it down and metabolize it. The form that it takes during this process appears to be as important as how much estrogen you consume and what type of exposure there is to your breasts. What you eat, what supplements you take, and the chemicals you are exposed to all have a major effect on your health, in this case your breasts. If you are estrogen dominant, several supplements are available that will help lower the level of estrogen in your body.

Diet plays a major role when it comes to breast problems. Certain foods have been known to increase the risk of pain and cyst formation in the breasts. Caffeine is well known to increase breast tenderness and the formation of cysts. Cut out caffeine from your diet and watch your breasts become softer.

Many of the meats from hormone-fed animals will increase estrogen levels in your body and cause more breast tenderness to occur. Even dairy products from animals given hormones will put excess hormones in your system. That is why it is important to use organic, hormone-free milk and cheeses whenever possible, and to eat hormone-free meat.

Besides being chock-full of antioxidant vitamins and minerals, fresh fruits and vegetables contain fiber to keep the colon working properly. When there is a good amount of fiber in the diet, estrogens that are excreted in the bile are then eliminated rapidly without the chance of reabsorbtion. This also facilitates the removal of other chemicals and toxins that the body is trying to clear.

In our very toxic world, there are thousands of invisible chemicals in our air, water, and food. Every year we consume pounds of these chemicals, which the liver then has to metabolize in order to eliminate. Many of these chemicals are similar in structure to estrogens and use the same enzymes for their elimination. This is another way in which estrogen levels can become higher: They compete with these chemicals for elimination.

There are specific supplements that assist the liver in clearing estrogens, as well as some of these pesticides. Calcium d-glucarate, a form of glucaric acid, enhances the body's ability to bind up estrogens and remove them from the body. It is nontoxic and is found in many foods including oranges, apples, broccoli, Brussels sprouts, and cabbage. If you have breast tenderness before your menses or premenopause, try taking 500 mg of calcium d-glucarate several times a day until the symptoms resolve.

Indole 3-carbinol and its active metabolite, DIM (di-indole-methane), are naturally found in cruciferous vegetables such as cabbage, broccoli, Brussels sprouts, and cauliflower. DIM has been shown to slow the growth of breast cancer cells and even cause cells to self-destruct. Read more about the cancer-protective effects of these supplements in Chapter 9.

In addition to these, formulas that help the liver break down fats, known as lipotrophic factors, are an excellent way to keep estrogen levels from going too high. The formulas contain a combination of choline, inositol, beet root extract, dandelion root, milk thistle, vitamins B_{12} and B_6, and betaine HCl. If you have symptoms of estrogen dominance such as breast tenderness or cysts, heavy bleeding, or ovarian cysts or fibroids, use these supplements to keep your estrogen levels low.

Alcohol

Besides being high in calories, alcohol is a fat. The same enzymes that help break down alcohol also break down estrogen. This breakdown requires specific amino acids, B vitamins, and minerals. Higher alcohol intake has been associated with higher levels of estrogen in the blood. For women using hormone replacement or oral contraceptives, levels of estrogen in the blood will increase when they consume alcohol. It has been shown that women with a high alcohol intake and low folate intake are at increased risk for breast cancer.

The higher levels of estrogen lead to tender and dense breasts. Research studies have found that women who consume more alcohol have denser breast tissue. Several animal studies have shown that alcohol may increase the spread of cancer cells in the body. Alcohol also increases the production of free radicals and causes oxidative stress on a cellular level. This damages cell membranes and DNA, and could result in the expression of cancer genes.

Cutting down on alcohol intake is thus important to prevent breast density changes and cancer. Whether you are still menstruating or in menopause—and especially if you are on HRT—keep your alcohol intake down to one drink daily. If you are drinking, make sure you are getting a good supply of vitamins and minerals.

CHAPTER 7

STRONG AND HEALTHY BONES

One of the most important things a woman can do to maintain her health is keep her bones strong. Osteoporosis is considered one of the silent killers for women: By the time a woman realizes that she has osteoporosis, she has lost so much bone mass that her bones are brittle and break easily. Hip and spinal fractures are painful and debilitating, They often lead to long-term illness and pain, as well as life-threatening problems such as pneumonia or blood clots.

Osteoporosis is difficult to treat once a large amount of bone loss has occurred, but it is entirely preventable. Risk factors for osteoporosis include early menopause, anorexia, overuse of steroids, high-protein diets, hyperthyroidism, mineral deficiencies, and family history. If you are Caucasian and have small bones, you have an increased risk of osteoporosis. Smoking will also cause bone loss to occur.

Check Your Bone Density

One of the greatest tools we have for preventing osteoporosis is the bone density test. This test sends a light wave into the bone and records the reflection. By reading what reflects back, you can determine how dense your bones are.

Getting this test in your forties and maybe even earlier can be helpful. It is good to see if you are someone who has not reached peak bone mass. Having this information before you actually go into menopause can give you motivation to work on building bone while you are still producing your own natural hormones.

Many women do not reach peak bone mass but don't find this out until they are in menopause. At that point, their main goal is to prevent further bone loss. Bone loss can occur long before menopause and becomes accelerated in the first five years after the menses stop. Irregular cycles, anorexia, chronic dieting, and even pregnancy can also increase the risk of bone loss in young women. Low levels of progesterone have been associated with lack of bone growth, as well.

Prevention is your best defense against this disease. Early detection and making lifestyle and dietary changes are the best ways to prevent broken bones in your later years.

It Takes More than Just Calcium

Every woman knows that it is important to eat calcium-rich foods and to take calcium to keep her bones strong. But bones are made up of a lot more than just calcium.

Bones contain many other minerals and require trace minerals for their synthesis. Magnesium is one of the minerals essential for healthy bones. Bones with more magnesium form smaller, irregular crystals that attach more firmly to one another. This can potentially make the bones more flexible than bones without as much magnesium.

Magnesium is also important for muscles, especially the heart. It is the one mineral that helps with energy production and is a cofactor in many enzyme reactions. In addition, it benefits the adrenal glands—the organs most important in responding to stress.

Blood tests can measure levels of calcium and magnesium in the blood. It is important to look at these levels carefully. Low normal levels can be indicative of a deficiency. Certain hormones will keep the blood levels stable and pull minerals from the tissues, muscles, and bones. Magnesium is found in higher concentrations inside cells, so there can be a severe deficiency before it shows up as a low magnesium level in the blood.

A test for intracellular mineral levels can be more accurate than testing the levels in the serum. Measuring a red blood cell mineral level can do this. A red blood cell mineral test is a regular blood test that measures levels of the mineral from inside the red blood cell. These tests can check more that just magnesium. Levels of zinc, copper, potassium, selenium, manganese, boron, and molybdenum are available with these tests. See the reference section at the end of this book for laboratories that perform these tests.

If the level of calcium in your blood that is less than 8.5, or you have a magnesium level less than 2.0, you could have low tissue levels of these minerals. The recommended daily allowance (RDA) for calcium for menopausal women is 1,000–1,500 mg. Too much calcium can be dangerous, for the calcium can accumulate in tissues, arteries, and joints. Kidney stones can form if you are consuming too much calcium and not drinking enough water. If you are concerned about your calcium absorption, have your doctor perform a twenty-four-hour urine test for calcium.

The RDA for magnesium is 300–450 mg. Many vitamin supplements lack adequate magnesium. Excess magnesium will cause diarrhea. Exercise and excess sweating, as well as intake of caffeinated beverages, will increase your daily requirement of magnesium.

Essential Nutrients for Healthy Bones

Other trace minerals required for healthy bones include zinc, copper, manganese, and boron. The modern diet tends to be deficient in these trace minerals, so a good supplement is necessary. Vitamin D, vitamin k, and even vitamin C are essential for healthy bones.

In a published study, women who were postmenopausal and not on estrogen experienced an increase in bone mass after taking a calcium/trace mineral combination, whereas women who took calcium alone continued to lose bone.

There are several supplements that contain these trace minerals along with calcium. To maintain strong bones, it is recommended that you take at least 1,000 mg of calcium and 500 mg of magnesium daily. Look for a supplement that contains additional minerals such as zinc, boron, and manganese in trace amounts.

Even essential fatty acids are considered important for the development of healthy bones. Without these oils, the bones will be more brittle—just as hair and nails become more brittle when these essential fatty acids are lacking in the diet.

Vitamin D is a fat-soluble vitamin that is required for the absorption of calcium through the intestines. It is considered the "sunshine vitamin," since it is synthesized in the skin upon exposure to sunlight. When supplementation with vitamin D is combined with calcium, the rate of hip fracture decreases. Vitamin D is toxic in high dosages, but 400–1,000 IU can be taken without risk.

Exercise for Life

There is no dispute about the importance of exercise. Research studies on the elderly have shown that even an exercise program initiated in people over sixty can have benefits. Exercise is essential to maintain bone mass. With exercise, the bone receives signals to regenerate.

The other major benefit of exercise is the strengthening of the muscles and tissues around the bone. When these muscles are more developed, they can offer greater support to the bones. There will be less chance of an injury with a fall when the muscles can provide strength and support.

The best form of exercise is weight-bearing exercise such as walking or jogging. Yoga is also excellent, since it especially strengthens the muscles of the upper body.

Exercise has many health benefits besides helping to keep your bones strong. It is important for the heart, circulation, and blood vessels. It helps lower blood pressure. It improves cholesterol readings by raising your levels of HDL—the good cholesterol.

When your muscles are strong, you will have a faster metabolism and less difficulty maintaining your weight. Exercise is a natural antidepressant and aphrodisiac. Women who have incorporated regular exercise into their lives report that they are happier, sleep better, and feel sexier.

Regular exercise will make you feel better about your body and be more confident about how you look—and it'll help you perform better during sex. There are a lot of reasons to get regular exercise besides just keeping your bones strong.

Bones and Hormones

For years we have known that estrogen is one of the best ways to protect against osteoporosis. This has certainly been proven in numerous studies. In fact, many women are taking estrogen on the advice of their physician to prevent osteoporosis. Progesterone is also involved in the growth of new bone. For some women, using progesterone alone may be enough to protect against bone loss.

Testosterone is another hormone that is important for maintaining bone density. Including small amounts of testosterone in the hormone formula—or for some women combining testosterone with just progesterone—will keep the bones strong.

If you are taking hormones to prevent bone loss, they will only work as long as you are taking them. This means you will need to take them for your lifetime. It is important to incorporate the other suggestions in this chapter rather than to rely solely on hormone therapy as your savior. Taking hormones isn't the only answer.

A more holistic approach is needed to prevent bone loss as you age. Incorporate lots of nutrient-rich foods in your diet. Find a form of exercise that you enjoy, and make it a part of your regular schedule. Take supplements to maintain the mineral and vitamin levels appropriate for your lifestyle and habits. Spend some time outdoors to make sure you are getting enough vitamin D, or make sure it is incorporated in the supplements you take. Remember, these bones need to last you a lifetime.

CHAPTER 8

A HEALTHY HEART

The risk of heart disease increases in women as they enter into menopause. The regular production of estrogen and progesterone during menstruation has a protective effect on circulation. The decline of these hormones is responsible for changes in blood vessels and blood flow.

The other effect of hormones is on cholesterol. Many women notice a change in their cholesterol level as they go into menopause. Women in menopause will often experience a fall in HDL (the good cholesterol) and a rise in LDL (the bad one) no matter how careful they are with their diet.

As women age, their risk of developing heart disease or atherosclerosis increases dramatically. Among women over sixty-five, heart disease is one of the leading causes of death. Until recently, it was thought that hormone replacement would provide protection from heart and cardiovascular changes for women after menopause. The recent releases of data from the HERS Study and the Women's Health Initiative have shown just the opposite, however: The use of conjugated estrogen with progestin did not protect against cardiovascular disease. In fact, there was an increase in the formation of the blood clots that can cause pulmonary embolism and strokes.

The biggest problem with this study is that only one hormone product was tested. Prempro, the product in question, contains conjugated estrogens and a synthetic progesterone, medroxyprogesterone. The natural bio-identical hormones in low dosages may not have the same risks.

One study on cholesterol showed that when natural micronized progesterone was used, HDL changes were more favorable than was seen with synthetic progestins. If this is the case, then there may be some benefit to using natural hormones biologically identical to their synthetic forms. Until there are more long-term studies on the use of these hormones, however, we will not know the answer to this question.

Reduce Your Risk

One of the major risk factors in heart disease is one you can do very little about: family history. It's true that you can't change your genes. What you *can* do is modulate your lifestyle and habits to affect the expression of your genes.

Other risks include an elevated LDL cholesterol, a low HDL cholesterol, diabetes, high blood pressure, lack of exercise, obesity (especially with excess weight in the abdomen), smoking, and elevated homocysteine. Many of these risks can be reduced or even eliminated through lifestyle changes.

Cholesterol and the Heart

Ever since it was discovered that elevated cholesterol increased the risk of atherosclerosis and heart disease, people have been watching their cholesterol. Over the years, the recommended levels have been lowered. Currently, it is considered best to keep your total cholesterol below 200, and your LDL below 130—or even below 100 if you have heart disease or any other risk factors. HDL should be at least thirty-five and preferably higher.

Cholesterol is manufactured in the liver. It is required for the production of hormones. All of the steroid hormones, including estrogen, progesterone, testosterone, and cortisol, are made from cholesterol. LDL cholesterol—it stands for "low-density lipoprotein"—has a higher concentration of cholesterol bound with a protein. These molecules are carried from the liver to the fat cells, and are thought to be responsible for plaque's narrowing the walls of the arteries.

HDL, or "high-density lipoprotein," carries cholesterol from the fat cells to the liver to be utilized. This molecule is protective against heart disease. A higher level is beneficial.

One of the other major theories that cholesterol is such a risk factor is inflammation. When inflammatory substances attach the blood vessels, an injury occurs. The cholesterol molecules then get caught in the reaction to form plaque. When plaque builds up, the arteries become thick and lose their flexibility.

Keeping cholesterol low will prevent the formation of plaque. Many doctors are using statin drugs to lower cholesterol. It is also believed that these drugs might have an anti-inflammatory effect, which further helps prevent atherosclerosis.

These drugs are very effective, but they do have side effects. Besides causing problems with the liver, statin drugs cause abdominal pain, bloating, and muscle aches. Statin drugs also reduce the production of coenzyme Q_{10}. Even for people who are watching their diet, genetic factors can cause increased cholesterol production. If you have tried everything to lower your cholesterol and have found yourself needing to take a statin drug, add a supplement of coenzyme Q_{10} to your daily regimen.

Another cause of high cholesterol is hypothyroidism, a condition in which the thyroid is not producing enough hormone. There are many factors behind hypothyroidism, but if you have high cholesterol and cannot find any explanation in your diet, make sure to have your thyroid levels checked.

Lower Cholesterol Naturally

If you do not want to take a statin drug, there may be other alternatives. Niacin (vitamin B_3) has been used to lower cholesterol. Large doses of 500–3,000 mg of niacin are required to lower cholesterol levels. Unfortunately, this can cause a severe flushing reaction, so it is important to start with smaller doses and build up. Another side effect of niacin therapy is elevated liver enzymes. A blood test should be done in the first few months of treatment to monitor liver enzymes. Sustained-release niacin is associated with a higher liver toxicity.

A natural form of statin drug is available as a red yeast rice extract. This supplement is not as strong as its prescription form and does not cause the same severity of side effects. Several companies offer this product; one combines a small amount of coenzyme Q_{10} with the red yeast rice extract. If you have mildly elevated cholesterol, this milder form may be helpful.

Guggul, an herb from the ayurvedic tradition, has also been reported to lower cholesterol. Studies have shown that guggul can lower serum cholesterol, LDL, and even triglycerides. Its effect on HDL is unclear. The dosage of guggul would be 100–500 mg daily. Side effects such as headaches and stomach upset could occur.

Guggul can also affect the thyroid by increasing production of thyroid stimulating hormone. If you are taking thyroid medication, have your levels measured—you may need to lower your dosage. Guggul could interact with some medications, such as propranolol and diltiazem.

Another supplement recently released to lower cholesterol is policosanol from an extract of sugarcane. Policosanol has been shown to inhibit the production of cholesterol in the liver and to increase the breakdown of LDL cholesterol. It is also effective in helping increase circulation in patients with intermittent claudication, and improving blood flow in patients with poor circulation in the heart.

Intermittent Claudication
A medical condition in which circulation to the lower extremities is reduced and an activity such as walking causes pain.

One of the mechanisms for this is the ability of policosanol to reduce platelet aggregation, or the stickiness of platelets. In one study, 20 mg of policosanol was found to be equivalent to 100 mg of

Platelet Aggregation
The phenomenon of platelets clumping together, making the blood thicker, slowing circulation, and causing the cells to get inadequate oxygen.

aspirin in reducing platelet aggregation. Policosanol and guggul can be used together.

Heart-Strengthening Herbs

Many women have heart-related symptoms when their hormones begin to change. They often experience chest discomfort, feel light-headed or dizzy, or have a pounding or irregular heartbeat. Often they will see a cardiologist, who will not find heart disease—but hopefully will recommend a hormone check. The exact reason for all of these symptoms is unknown except that lowered levels of estrogen, progesterone, and testosterone will often affect circulation and the autonomic nervous system.

For those women with mild symptoms that don't require medication, herbal supplements may be helpful. Two herbs can be especially beneficial to the heart: crataegus and motherwort.

Crataegus, also known as hawthorn berry, is one of the most popular herbs in Europe for the heart. The berries and leaves are very high in bioflavonoids and procyanidins, which are very good for circulation and healthy blood vessels. Crataegus can be used to lower blood pressure and improve the function of a weakening heart muscle in heart failure. Because crataegus interacts with cardiovascular drugs, it should only be used under the advice of your doctor. If your symptoms are mild enough not to require medication, you might try 200–500 mg of hawthorn powder two to three times daily.

Motherwort (*Leonuri cardiaca*) is used for calming and strengthening the heart. It is known to reduce anxiety and palpitations, especially when associated with hot flashes. Motherwort has a direct effect on slowing the heart rate and reducing spasms. It also reduces platelet aggregation and thins the blood. It can be combined with crataegus but should not be

combined with other herbs that contain cardiac glycosides such as digitalis. Drink a cup of motherwort
tea by steeping $1/2$ teaspoon of the leaves and flower
buds in a cup of water, or use up to 2 grams of the
dried powder daily.

Antioxidants and the Heart

Antioxidants are known to improve cellular function
and protect against free-radical damage. One of the
main theories behind damage to the heart and arteries attributes it to excess free radicals from various
different sources. There are several different vitamins
and nutrients that work together to provide antioxidant protection to the cells.

There have been numerous studies of the effects
of vitamin E supplements on the heart and other
forms of vascular disease. Besides having an antioxidant effect, vitamin E also helps keep platelets from
sticking together. Many of the studies have shown
a favorable effect on both coronary artery disease
and atherosclerosis. The Nurses' Health Study found
that women taking more than 100 IU of vitamin E enjoyed a 44 percent reduction in major coronary artery
disease.

Lipoic acid is a powerful antioxidant that works
together with vitamin E to potentiate its effect.
Although long-term studies of vitamin E and alpha-
lipoic acid on the heart are not available, combining
these nutrients has been shown to offer more powerful antioxidant protection than either one alone. A
dose of 400 IU can be combined with 100 mg of
alpha-lipoic acid.

Because many diets are deficient in antioxidants,
and because environmental stresses have increased
our exposure to free-radical damage, supplementation with a formula rich in antioxidants is your best
protection.

B Vitamins and Heart Disease

Another risk factor for heart disease was recently
discovered. A specific gene variation can cause an

increase in homocysteine. Elevated levels of homo-cysteine will facilitate the development of vascular disease by causing damage to blood vessels. This damage can also affect the brain and increase the risk of Alzheimer's disease and dementia. When B vitamins are deficient—especially folic acid, B_6, and B_{12}—excess homocysteine forms. These elevated levels can be measured in the blood. Lowering levels of homocysteine by taking a supplement with those vitamins will reduce the development of plaque in the arteries.

In a Swiss heart study, 553 patients with heart dis-ease were double-blinded after an angioplasty pro-cedure to receive a B-vitamin supplement containing 1 mg of folic acid, 400 mg of vitamin B_{12}, and 10 mg of vitamin B_6. Each patient was treated for six months. There was a significant decrease in the need for a repeat angioplasty and other cardiac complications in the group treated with the B vitamins. The authors concluded in the study that B vitamins are beneficial for patients with heart disease.

To find out if you are getting enough B vitamins to keep your homocysteine levels low, ask your doc-tor to do a simple blood test to check your levels. It is important to keep these levels low to prevent heart disease and stroke. If you have elevated levels of homocysteine, a vitamin supplement with B vitamins can be a lifesaver.

Inflammation and the Heart

C reactive Protein

A protein pro-duced as a result of nonspecific inflammation in the body.

Another important marker has been found to accelerate the development of heart disease: C reactive protein. It is produced by the liver in response to infection, inflammation, or injured tissue. Research has shown that, es-pecially for women, an elevated level of this protein in the blood is associ-ated with an increase in the risk of heart disease despite normal levels of cholesterol.

An elevation of C reactive protein may be due to

some type of low-grade infection, such as an overgrowth of bacteria in the intestine, or it may have to do with certain foods in the diet. A blood test can determine if you have an elevated C reactive protein.

If you are showing elevated C reactive protein, many doctors are recommending the use of statin drugs. Another approach is to supplement with omega-3 fish oils. These oils have a powerful anti-inflammatory effect on the body, as well as many other health benefits.

A Happy Heart

Of course, the heart is also a major center for emotions and feelings. Feelings of sadness, depression, and stress will affect the heart. Many times, life situations can be difficult and no matter what we do, we can't help feeling these emotions. It is normal with many of the pressures in life to experience periods of feeling depressed, sad, or anxious. What we do during those times and how we handle them will make a difference in what effects they might have on our body.

To keep your heart happy if you are going through a rough time in life, it is important to start paying more attention to yourself. You may be having pressures at work or at home. First, be aware that feelings are better felt than repressed. Find someone you can talk to about what is going on—a friend, your family doctor, and perhaps a therapist if warranted.

Do something special for yourself, even if it is something small. Make it something that will bring you joy. Buy yourself a bouquet of flowers. Watch a funny movie. Take a walk in the woods or at the beach. Being in nature will often help you feel calm again.

Remember to love yourself no matter what is happening. Love is the emotion that heals the heart. Sometimes it's hard to do this when you are going through a tough time. Ask for help from family and friends to remember this.

Do five minutes of deep breathing or yoga to help relax. Restart that meditation process you've forgotten. In your meditation, visualize the problem resolved. Get out with friends or do something that will take your mind off your problems, even if it is for just a short time. Keeping the heart healthy means also working with your soul. It's a constant process, so learn to check in with yourself from time to time in your busy life to see how you are feeling.

Save Your Heart

Since heart disease and stroke are among the leading causes of death for women after menopause, it is important to pay attention not only to how you live your life but also to symptoms. Many women with heart problems do not have typical symptoms of acute chest pain. They may have milder or unusual symptoms. Because of this, they are often not diagnosed appropriately.

Most of the risk factors for heart disease are preventable with changes in your lifestyle. Diabetes and high blood pressure can increase the risk of developing atherosclerosis. Keep your blood pressure under good control and pay attention to your diet. Many people are resistant to taking medication, but uncontrolled high blood pressure will contribute to problems with the heart and vascular system. There are many newer choices for medications with fewer side effects, if you need to take them. Regular exercise and a healthy diet are especially important if you have risk factors for heart disease.

Syndrome X
A metabolic condition characterized by abdominal obesity, elevated blood lipids, high blood pressure, and insulin resistance.

If you are diabetic, monitor your blood sugar and watch your diet. High blood sugar will increase the development of plaque in the arteries. Increases in insulin from overeating carbohydrates are associated with Syndrome X. This condition features an excess of insulin associated with obesity and high blood pressure. This rise in blood pressure will increase your risk of heart disease and stroke.

Smoking is one of the greatest contributors to heart disease. Many people are aware of the fact that smoking increases the risk of cancer—especially lung cancer—but smoking also accelerates the development of heart disease and will increase your chances of heart attack and stroke. It is very difficult for some people to stop smoking, but with the medication Zyban and nicotine patches or lozenges, many people have been able to do so.

Eat a healthy diet with lots of fresh fruits and vegetables. Take supplements that contain B vitamins, calcium and magnesium, antioxidants, and fish oils to give your cells the extra nourishment they need. Get regular exercise. Exercise will increase cells' efficiency at using oxygen and improve circulation. If you have been having more stress in your life, start a meditation program. Find ways to get the support that you need. It's all about keeping your heart healthy—and you'll see the benefits in other areas of your life, as well.

CHAPTER 9

CANCER PREVENTION FOR A LIFETIME

Cancer is a complex disease that has more than one cause. Despite all of the millions of dollars poured into research on prevention and treatment, cancer remains one of the leading causes of death for women. There are hundreds of different types of cancer; even within one organ, such as the breast, several different forms of cancer can occur that have different patterns, growth cycles, and treatments. Although breast cancer is one of the most common cancers for women, it isn't one of the leading causes of cancer deaths. There are more women dying from lung cancer than any other cause. Colon, cervical, uterine, and ovarian cancers are the other more common cancers occurring in women.

Since we do not know the exact cause of cancer, it is difficult to approach prevention with any certainty. There are, however, many theories about how cancer develops. From these theories, we can make changes in our lives that over time may reduce our risk of cancer.

Certainly early detection via mammograms, ultrasounds, Pap smears, and colonoscopies can find cancers early enough to make them curable. Over the past ten years, the numbers of cancer survivors have increased dramatically due to early detection and treatment. Yet we still ask the question: *Can we prevent cancer—and if so, how?*

What Causes Cancer?

Cancer is a disease of multiple causes. It is believed

to be due to a combination of factors, including heredity and the environment. Specific genes have been identified that control the growth of cells. One single mutation in these genes can be enough to play a role in the development of cancer. A change in DNA can cause a mutation that will send the cells growing out of control.

This mutation can be caused by free-radical damage, which is occurring in overwhelming numbers due to changes in our environment. Pollution, radiation, toxic chemicals, pesticides, viruses, alcohol, heavy metals, and even excess exercise all have the potential to cause cell damage. Particularly with breast cancer, exposure to pesticides has been considered a risk.

Pesticides are fat soluble and can collect in breast tissue. Counties where hazardous wastes sites are found are 6.5 times more likely to have elevated rates of breast cancer. Pesticides such as DDT, PCBs, and DDE have been found concentrated in breast tumors. Currently, more than thirty thousand chemicals in our environment are untested.

Normally, the cell has systems in place to protect itself against free-radical damage and repair damaged DNA. When the cell has lost the ability to repair these damaged cells and the immune system fails to destroy them, however, cancer can develop. Excess exposure to toxins plus a lack of nutrients will weaken the cell's ability to repair the damaged DNA. Vitamins and minerals are essential to keep these systems functioning.

Excess exposure to estrogens is another factor involved in the development of cancer. According to Malcolm Pike, Ph.D., contemporary women have an increased lifetime exposure to estrogen since they have hundreds more ovulation cycles than did our hunter-gatherer foremothers. Modern women are delaying childbirth and are having fewer pregnancies. Hormones in meats and dairy products also will increase a woman's exposure to estrogen. A definite increase in estrogen dominance has been noted in the general population, with the associated frequency of problems such as fibroids, ovarian cysts, and endometriosis. Obesity is another factor that will increase the lifetime risk of cancer, since fat cells produce estrogens.

Taking the estrogen theory even farther: As they are metabolized, specific forms of estrogen appear to be stronger and present more of a risk than others. When estrogens are broken down, several types of estrones are formed. The 16-OH estrone and 4-OH estrone have an increased carcinogenic effect on the cell, whereas the 2-OH estrone appears to reduce the growth of cancer cells.

In a research study of 10,786 premenopausal women, those women with higher 2-OH estrone levels were 40 percent less likely to develop breast cancer during the five years of the study. There are numerous factors that influence how the body produces these estrogen metabolites. Cruciferous vegetables (broccoli, cabbage, and so forth), for instance, contain substances that increase the amount of the more protective estrogens.

Another study from the Norris Cancer Center at the University of Southern California compared these same estrogens in postmenopausal women with breast cancer against a control group. Researchers measured the levels of estrones in the urine and did not find the same high levels of 16-OH estrone in breast cancer patients. This study was much smaller than the one described above, however, and was on postmenopausal women.

Oncogenes
Genes that encourage the growth of normal cells but that, when mutated or overexpressed, can lead to the growth of cancer.

One more factor is the production of the catechol estrogens. A process called methylation in the liver breaks down these estrogens. When there are too many 4-catechol estrogens or not enough enzymes available to break them down, a quinone estrogen forms. These quinone estrogens cause mutations in DNA that increase the expression of oncogenes and tumor suppressor genes.

Free radicals can lead to an excess production of these estrogens. B vitamins and magnesium are needed to help metabolize these estrogens and prevent them from becoming quinones. So it is a combination of the overproduction of and inability to properly clear these substances that will potentially increase the risk of cancer cells to occur.

Changes in the cell's metabolism can alter the enzymes available for clearing these toxins. Diets low in protein and essential fatty acids and high in sugar will further reduce the body's ability to detoxify these substances. Vitamin and mineral deficiencies limit the amount of detoxification the body can handle. As you see, it is not one single factor that causes these changes, but a combination that will predispose cells to become cancerous.

Lower Your Estrogen Exposure

Can we lower our estrogen exposure? Yes, there are actions you can take to lower your risk of exposure to excess estrogen. Making changes in your diet and adding specific nutritional supplements have been found to be helpful in keeping estrogen levels low and preventing the excess production of quinones.

The diet described in Chapter 6—high in fiber, fruits, and vegetables—will give you all the nutrients your body needs. Fiber allows estrogen to be bound and eliminated via the colon. Fiber also feeds the bacteria in the intestine that prevent estrogen from being reabsorbed into the bloodstream.

Two other supplements can further protect against elevated estrogens: calcium d-glucarte and indole 3-carbinol. Glucaric acid is a naturally occurring compound found in apples, oranges, broccoli, cabbage, and potatoes. It enhances liver detoxification and elimination of estrogen. As a supplement, it is available as calcium d-glucarate. In animal studies, it has been shown to lower estradiol levels and inhibit the development of cancer. It is nontoxic and has no side effects. As a supplement, doses of 2–3 grams several times daily can be used for symptoms of excess estrogen.

Indole 3-carbinol is also found in cruciferous vegetables such as cabbage, broccoli, and cauliflower. In numerous studies, I 3 C was effective in preventing cancers. One of the actions of I 3 C is to alter the metabolism of estrones by encouraging the 2-OH estrone and reducing the amount of 16-OH estrone. The most common dosage for women is 400 mg daily. Another form of I 3 C is available as di-indole-methane (DIM). DIM is a more stable form of the I 3 C and is also available as a supplement. The dosage is 75 mg of active DIM daily.

A test can be done to see if you are creating an excess amount of these estrogens. The levels of 2-OH estrone and 16-OH estrone can be measured in urine and blood. Great Smokies Diagnostic Laboratory and Metametrix have test kits available to check these levels and determine if using a supplement will be helpful.

Cancer Prevention

The most preventable causes of cancer are lifestyle and diet. Even with a genetic predisposition to cancer, it takes something to initiate the abnormal DNA to express itself. Currently, it is believed that only 5 to 10 percent of all cancers are genetic in origin. Smoking, for example, increases the risk of lung cancer, and also breast cancer, cervical cancer, and many others. Smoke increases the production of free radicals that overwhelm the cell and lead to damaged DNA.

Nutrition plays a major role when it comes to cancer. A study published in the *British Journal of Biomedical Sciences* in 1994 of sixty-two patients in the early stages of active cancer found substantial deficiencies. These patients had low intakes of vitamins A, C, and E, as well as essential vitamins and minerals. In another study from the American Dietary Association, deficiencies in beta-carotene, vitamin

B_6, folic acid, and zinc were associated with a lowered immune response and greater risk of developing cancer.

According to Bruce Ames, Ph.D., one of the leading researchers on genetic mutations and cancer, we are exposed to thousands of carcinogens that are both natural and synthetic. The environment is so infused with chemicals that it is impossible to avoid them. Even people who eat totally organically were found to have more than a hundred carcinogens in their bodies.

Our primary defense against cancer caused by such exposures is nutrition. Supplements such as folic acid, vitamins C and E, and zinc play a role in the detoxification of chemicals, as well as the protection of DNA from mutations. Lipoic acid has been shown to reduce DNA damage to cells exposed to radiation. For the best protection, take a high-quality supplement with antioxidants, as well as eating a diet rich in these nutrients.

Emotions and Cancer

There is no question that disease often arises during periods of high emotional stress. Cancer is no different. Many patients whom I have cared for told me that they had experienced emotional stress prior to the development of cancer. Emotional stress weakens the immune system and makes a person more susceptible to cancer or other illnesses. Although we cannot avoid having emotional difficulties in life, we can change how we handle them.

Repressed emotions such as anger, resentment, or fear create blockages that affect our health. There are many tools available for getting in touch with these buried emotions and releasing them. One of the best ways to stay healthy is to create a system to check in with yourself and learn to feel and express emotional pain.

Our society has created lots of ways to repress and ignore the value of emotions. Instead of feeling and acknowledging emotional pain, we take drugs, drink alcohol, or create diversions to block feelings. We are emotional beings, however, and learning to feel our emotions and express them is a very powerful experience.

For healing to take place on any level, we need to get in touch with our inner thoughts, feelings, and desires. This can be done with a variety of techniques, from psychotherapy to guided meditation and releasing techniques such as the Sedona Method. With cancer—as with any illness—there are spiritual dimensions to the healing process.

Getting in touch with repressed feelings is the first step. Experiencing love and forgiveness toward yourself and others is the next. The inner peace that comes from this will facilitate the healing process. If you are suffering from an illness, it may not be easy to get to the emotional issues and feelings buried in your unconscious. Get help from a good counselor or therapist who is experienced in helping people with chronic disease.

CHAPTER 10

Sexual Vitality after Menopause

Sex is an important part of a relationship. With sexual intimacy, we connect with our partner in a loving way. Sex relaxes us and produces endorphins that help us reduce the effects of stress on our body. A twenty-five-year follow-up study on aging published in 1982 found that women who had regular sex and enjoyed it lived longer. In that same study, the men who had increased frequency of sexual intercourse also enjoyed greater longevity.

When women enter into premenopause and menopause, their hormone levels fall. As this happens, there will often be a change in libido and the quality of sex. Many women can have difficulty with lubrication or achieving orgasm. They often lose their interest in sex, even in happy relationships.

As many ways as women are different, there will be differences in how women adjust to these lower levels in their sex drive. There used to be a belief in the medical community that when women went into menopause, they would have a better sex life since they wouldn't have to worry about birth control. Now with more awareness, we are finding out that many women have problems. They need and want help.

Sarah was forty-two when she came to see me. She had been treated with chemotherapy for Hodgkin's lymphoma and was still having regular periods. The past year had been very stressful for her, and she was starting to have symptoms of premenopause. She was getting hot at night, but even more importantly, she had lost her sex drive. She was in a new relationship, she loved her partner, but she just didn't have the same desire she used to. Her doctor had tested her FSH but it was normal. There was nothing wrong with her, her doctor had said.

Help—My Hormones Are Falling

Some women, like Sarah, will start to experience lowered hormone levels even in their early forties. Sarah had also been treated with chemotherapy and had a very stressful year. All of these things affected her hormones, and lower hormone levels can mean changes in mood and sexual performance. When we measured her hormone levels, she had no measurable testosterone and low levels of estrogen and progesterone.

As estrogen levels fall, vaginal tissues become thinner, pale, and lose lubrication and flexibility. Tissues become dry in general, with women often complaining of dry skin, dry eyes, and dryness vaginally. When estrogen levels become very low, the vagina can become smaller; penetration can be difficult and often impossible. Intercourse can be very painful.

Lower estrogen levels will also change the bacterial environment of the vagina and make a woman more susceptible to vaginal and urinary tract infections. Because estrogen helps keep the muscles that control urination in good tone, women can have problems with bladder control.

Testosterone and Desire

Androgen Deficiency
A deficiency in the production of androgen-type steroid hormones, such as testosterone and DHEA.

When testosterone levels become low, many women will begin to experience a lower sexual desire. Achieving orgasm can become more difficult. This condition of low testosterone is called androgen deficiency.

Some women will notice loss of sexual interest even in their thirties and forties. Our hormones and our sexual desire are closely connected.

Testosterone is the hormone of desire. We think of it as a male hormone, but women have testosterone at about one-tenth the level of a man. There are other, more systemic symptoms associated with low testosterone, including fatigue, depression, apathy, and loss of muscle mass and strength. Women may even feel difficulty with concentration or have trouble feeling excited about their lives.

Testosterone is made in small amounts in the adrenal glands but primarily by the ovaries. Women who have had their ovaries removed also suffer from low testosterone levels. Many doctors focus only on replacing estrogen and forget about looking at other hormones that might need to be replaced.

Problems with the adrenal glands will also cause testosterone levels to be low. Dehydro-epiandrosterone, a hormone that is made in the adrenal glands, is also made in small amounts by the ovaries. As it is metabolized, it becomes converted into testosterone and estrogen. Low DHEA levels are often seen when testosterone and estrogen levels are low.

Even birth control pills can cause testosterone levels to become low for several reasons. Birth control pills will lower the amount of testosterone produced by the ovaries, since they will stop the ovulation process and the usual production of hormones that goes along with it. When you take birth control pills, the liver produces more of a protein called sex hormone binding globulin (SHBG). This holds on to the hormones in the blood so that not the entire hormone is released to the cells. When levels of SHBG are high, more testosterone is bound up to this protein. There is less testosterone available to the cells, and a relative deficiency of testosterone develops. Some women will notice that they

Sex Hormone Binding Globulin SHBG)
A protein produced by the liver that binds to steroid hormones, thereby preventing large amounts of these hormones from circulating in the blood.

are fine during the week of placebo or no pills, but as soon as they start taking the pills their libido wanes.

Until recently, many doctors didn't recognize the importance of testosterone for a woman. In fact, natural testosterone even now is available only from compounding pharmacies. The other form of testosterone available for women is in the form of Estratest, a combination of methyltestosterone and conjugated estrogens. Methyltestosterone has a higher liver toxicity and should not be used in patients with a history of liver disease.

Women who have had their ovaries removed particularly benefit from replacement of testosterone. In a study at Massachusetts General Hospital, seventy-five women aged thirty-one to fifty-six who had their ovaries removed were randomized to receive either 0.15 or 0.3 mg of testosterone transdermally for twelve weeks. They were all treated with estrogens or additional testosterone. The higher testosterone dosage was associated with a two- to threefold increase in frequency of sexual activity and pleasure. The women treated with testosterone reported improved well-being and less depression. There were no reports of negative side effects such as acne or excess hair growth.

For women who have been treated for breast cancer, methyltestosterone might be a better choice, since it cannot be converted into estrogen. Methyltestosterone is available from compounding pharmacies in creams or sublingual lozenges.

If you are experiencing a gradual loss of sexual desire in an otherwise satisfying relationship, or persistent fatigue without a clear cause, ask you doctor to check your testosterone levels. Testosterone levels are higher in the morning and probably higher during the luteal phase, the second half of the menstrual cycle. It is important for men to measure the free level of testosterone, but for women measuring total testosterone levels is fine. It is less costly, and women's levels are much lower than men's; a lower level of total testosterone usually also means that the level of free testosterone is low.

For women with vaginal dryness, testosterone cream can be used several times a week to improve sexual response and lubrication. It is usually best to start with a low concentration such as 1–2 mg per gram of cream.

Herbal Aphrodisiacs

For women who prefer to avoid hormone therapy, there are many other herbal alternatives that keep sexual desire burning after menopause. As mentioned in Chapter 3, some herbal medicines are rich in phytoestrogens and other nutrients that will enrich hormone production. Other herbal remedies contain substances that help improve circulation into the vagina and increase lubrication.

Damiana is one of the best-known herbal aphrodisiacs for women. These small leaves from a shrub plant that grows in Texas and Mexico contain alkaloids that are thought to be hormonelike in their action. The exact components of damiana are unknown. It can be used as powder in capsules at a dosage of 1–4 grams daily, as a tea, or a liquid tincture.

Deer antler and maca root (both mentioned in Chapter 3) are wonderful herbs to boost libido. Both stimulate hormone production and also enhance endurance and strength, qualities needed for great sex. They can be taken in powder or capsules.

Muira puama, also known as potency wood, is native of the Amazon region. It historically has been used for men but now is being combined with other herbs for women. The components of this herb have not been well studied, but its action is said to help improve circulation into the pelvis and genitals.

Muira puama works well when combined with one of the hormone enhancers such as deer antler, maca, or ginseng. Since they have two different actions, they are synergistic when used together. There still is very limited information on this herb, but it is certainly one to be aware of as we learn more about its amazing sexual-enhancing potential.

Topical Creams

For those women who do not want to take oral estrogens, there are several creams and tablets that can be used in the vagina to reverse the problem of vaginal dryness. Estradiol is available by prescription as a cream and as Vagifem—the brand name of a small tablet that gets absorbed into the vagina. These can be inserted on an as-needed basis to keep the vaginal lining moist and soft. Estriol can be ordered by your physician in cream form to be used in the vagina. Several studies from Italy, Germany, and Japan have shown that estriol cream in the vagina is effective in reducing the dryness that occurs with menopause. In the United States, estriol is available from compounding pharmacies.

Testosterone cream is another wonderful product to help with vaginal dryness; it also enhances libido and orgasm. Have your doctor order this from a compounding pharmacy. It is usually best to start with a small concentration of 1–2 mg of testosterone per gram of cream. The cream can be applied to the vagina and clitoris as often as needed, but can be especially useful about an hour before intercourse.

Prescription hormone creams for the vagina will have some systemic absorption and may have some of the same side effects as when they are taken orally. With these creams, however, it is possible to use very small doses, and not to use them daily. Vagifem has a much lower absorption potential and has therefore been recommended for women who have had breast cancer. It does not appear to cause a thickening of the uterine lining, as some creams do.

For women who prefer not to use hormone creams, several over-the-counter products can be helpful. One of the ways that circulation increases into the vaginal area is by the neurotransmitter nitric oxide. This amazing substance is released from the amino acid arginine. Nitric oxide is also the mechanism behind Viagra and several other new medications to enhance sexual response that will be released soon. Various creams containing arginine have been shown to help improve blood flow into the vaginal area. They increase lubrication and enhance sexual response. Viagra can also be compounded into a topical cream for women who experience difficulty with orgasm or lubrication.

Nitric Oxide
A newly discovered neurotransmitter that causes dilation of blood vessels.

Before you try any of these creams during intercourse, do a test on a small area of the labia. (Some creams contain menthol or herbal extracts that may be irritating.) If you develop any irritation, be cautious. Astroglide is another product available in the pharmacy that is an excellent lubricant and is not irritating. Several companies offer creams with phytoestrogens that are mild and may help improve the vaginal lining. These creams contain extracts of black cohosh, red clover, and other plant-based estrogens. None of these products has been tested in large studies at this time.

Great Sex after Menopause

Yes, it is possible to have great sex after menopause. Knowing your body and what it takes to turn you on is the key. A woman should be aware of what her likes and dislikes are, what stimulates her and excites her. One of the benefits to growing older is that by the time you reach this stage of life, you're likely more comfortable with yourself.

Having great sex means knowing how to communicate with and teach your partner how to turn you on. Sexual partners, whether men or women, are not mind readers and may need a little coaching. Learning how to ask for what you want during sex is just as important as getting your hormonal balance going.

Make sex fun and playful. Be imaginative. Wear sexy lingerie, use sensual aromatic oils, or do a striptease. Take belly-dancing classes. Whatever it takes to let the sexual part of you come alive. My book *Love Potions* contains more information on ways to boost libido and enjoyment. Remember, regular sex is good for your health and vitality. It will keep your hormones going and may even help you live a longer, healthier life.

CHAPTER 11

A CLEAR MIND, EMOTIONS, AND THINKING

The effects of a woman's hormones on her mood and emotional state are very powerful. Hormone levels that are low, high, or simply out of balance can make a woman feel irritable, easily angered, anxious, weepy, or depressed. During the transition from premenopause into menopause, hormone levels will move from very high to very low. Many women will seek the help of a psychiatrist or therapist to find out why they are depressed or anxious. A well-trained mental health professional who sees such emotional swings will recommend having hormones tested, especially when the shifts occur with changes in the menstrual cycle.

Another major effect of falling hormones is on mental focus and memory. Short-term memory loss is a common issue that women notice as their hormone levels fall. Research has shown that women who have taken estrogen have fewer problems with dementia and Alzheimer's disease. If you are starting to notice a waning memory, there are many things you can do to keep your mind sharp besides taking estrogen.

Emotions and Hormones

During premenopause, women often have normal or high estrogen with lower-than-normal progesterone levels. This can cause not only irregular bleeding patterns but also mood swings, depending upon how high or low the levels are. When estrogen levels are high, you will retain water. This increase in fluid often causes the nervous system to feel more irritated.

Progesterone can have a calming effect on the nervous system. When estrogen levels are high and progesterone levels are low, you may feel more irritable. As a result, you might feel easily upset and angry over things that might not normally bother you.

As a women transitions into menopause, the levels of all hormones will fall. Progesterone, estrogen, and testosterone have a profound effect on mood. When estrogen levels and progesterone levels fall, emotions can range from feeling depressed and overwhelmed to being extremely anxious. Some women might even feel that life is too difficult and not worth living. If you are having these types of mood swings, this is definitely the time to have your hormones checked. Many therapists will prescribe antidepressants to help treat the symptoms, which may or may not be effective. Having your hormones checked is extremely important if you are having these difficulties.

Kathy came to see me crying, saying, "I'm so emotional, and I feel like I can't stop crying. Even little things that used to not bother me at all are making me so upset. I don't know what to do. I also haven't had a period for several months." After hearing about her missed periods, I knew that a hormone test was essential.

We found that Kathy's progesterone level was very low, but she had a normal estrogen level. Her FSH was 25. She was in the beginning stages of premenopause. She started on progesterone capsules 100 mg daily; within a week, her emotional symptoms had stabilized and she was feeling her old self again.

It is essential to have both estrogen and progesterone levels checked if you are having trouble, since each can be associated with severe depression and anxiety. When progesterone levels are low, you are more likely to feel depressed and weepy. During premenopause, the ovaries may not be releasing an egg every month and therefore will not be producing the same amount of progesterone as they once were.

Restoring progesterone to more normal levels can

be very helpful, and not only for a woman's emotional well-being. During these months of imbalances, with a high or normal estrogen and lower progesterone, a woman can become more prone to heavy bleeding that might require a D&C, or to ovarian cysts, fibroids, or breast problems. Replacing progesterone can be accomplished by using progesterone in capsules, sublingual drops, or cream. This will simulate a more normal cycle and prevent problems from excess estrogen.

D&C
A procedure also known as dilatation and curettage used to clean out the uterine lining to stop bleeding, and to evaluate the uterus for cancerous or precancerous cells.

Low Estrogen and Depression

As a woman moves into menopause, estrogen levels will fall. Besides experiencing hot flashes and sleep problems, some women are often prone to severe episodes of depression and anxiety. The exact reason why this happens is unclear, but it is thought that hormones affect serotonin receptors in the brain. The relationship between hormone levels and quality of life can be dramatic. For women with severe depression, using natural estrogen and progesterone will bring back a sense of calm and well-being, along with restoring sleep.

When mood swings are severe, using prescription dosages of hormones may be the best option to restore blood levels into the premenopausal range. Estradiol is available in oral tablets and can be compounded into the best dosage for you. Topical creams and patches also will deliver estrogen into the bloodstream and bypass the liver.

Because of the potential risks of estrogen, it is best to use the smallest dosage that you need and combine it with other hormones such as progesterone, testosterone, and DHEA. Replacement of hormones can be a lifesaver for women suffering from mood symptoms.

Androgen Deficiency Syndrome

Low levels of testosterone can affect libido but also have a profound effect on mood and energy level. When testosterone levels are low, a woman may experience more fatigue and low libido but also depression and apathy. This syndrome, now recognized as androgen deficiency, is more common than previously realized. Some women may even have normal levels of estrogen and progesterone, but very low levels of testosterone.

Testosterone replacement is being recommended for women with low levels of this hormone who are symptomatic. For women who are in menopause and taking estrogen and progesterone, adding a small amount of testosterone can also be helpful in boosting energy sex drive and mood.

Since testosterone production in the body is dependent upon zinc, making sure that you are getting enough of this mineral can be important. Several studies on men have shown that when zinc levels were restored to normal, testosterone levels also increased. You can check for zinc deficiency with a test for red blood cell zinc levels. To restore levels when they are low, supplement with 50 mg of zinc daily.

Boost Your Brain Naturally

One of the hormones best known as a memory aid is pregnenolone. This steroid-based hormone is one of the first substances to be synthesized from cholesterol as a precursor to the other steroid hormones such as progesterone, DHEA, cortisol, estrogen, and testosterone. It is also found in large amounts in nerve tissue, especially in the brain. In animal studies, the addition of pregnenolone was associated with improved cognitive function and memory.

Levels of pregnenolone can be measured in the blood. Restoring levels by taking a supplement may be the best way to activate a fading memory. If you have low levels, start with about 30 mg daily. Some women may require up to 100 mg for replacement to physiologic levels. Side effects such as anxiety or irritability can occur, so it is best to start with lower dosages and work up. Since pregnenolone can be stimulating, I usually recommend taking it in the morning.

Another hormone useful for its effect on the brain, mood, and memory is DHEA. This hormone is another one that appears to be found in large amounts in the central nervous system. With aging, the levels of this hormone decline. Studies on animals have shown that when rats were given DHEA, they increased the number of newly formed red blood cells. Replacement of DHEA in men and women has been associated with improvement of the immune system and mood. Women reported an improved sense of well-being and better sleep. As mentioned in Chapter 2, DHEA levels can be measured in the blood as DHEA-S.

Supplements of DHEA are available either over the counter or from compounding pharmacies. As with any supplement, be sure that you are purchasing from a reputable company that has good quality control, or have your compounding pharmacy make a custom dosage for you. For women, small dosages may be best to start with—say, 5–10 mg daily. Monitor your blood levels and be aware of side effects such as acne, breast tenderness, weight gain, and hair growth or loss.

Taking supplements of pregnenolone and DHEA may be helpful in reducing the amount of estrogen you need to take to control symptoms of menopause. There are no data on whether these hormones will provide other benefits such as increases in bone density or improved cholesterol ratios. Since they may increase the amount of estrogen and testosterone, use caution if you have had a hormone-sensitive cancer, and monitor your hormone levels by having your blood checked periodically.

Herbal Mood and Brain Boosters

Rhodiola rosea is a lovely root known as golden root

or rose root growing in the high-altitude, arctic regions of Europe and Asia. It has a long history of use in Russia and Scandinavia, where extensive research has also been done. It is an adaptogen like Siberian ginseng. Studies report that rhodiola can stabilize mood and improve the symptoms of anxiety and depression. It reduces stress and protects nerve and brain cells against free-radical damage. This amazing root will increase brain neurotransmitters to enhance mood, memory, and thinking.

Like ginseng, rhodiola has been used to prevent fatigue in athletes and reduce the effects of stress on the brain. It affects the endocrine system to improve the function of the thyroid and thymus glands, and has even helped improve sexual response. It does not contain phytoestrogens but may bind estrogen receptors. The exact reason for this is still unclear. This plant has a wide range of uses, and as more studies are done, there will be even more applications for it.

Rhodiola has very low toxicity, and no adverse side effects have been reported. It can be taken as a tincture or in powder form. The dosage is 50–100 mg two times daily. It can be combined with other herbs such as Siberian ginseng, American ginseng, or maca.

St. John's wort is a beautiful yellow flower that grows wild in Europe and the northern United States. Traditionally, it has been used for depression, anxiety, and pain. The active ingredients in St. John's wort are known to affect levels of serotonin and gamma-aminobutyric acid (GABA), as well as norepinephrine and dopamine. Several studies have shown that St. John's wort can be as effective as many of the prescription antidepressants. It is helpful for mild to moderate depression; for conditions of severe depression, more conventional approaches should be used.

Side effects of St. John's wort include allergic reactions, skin rashes, sun sensitivity, and stomach upset. It can affect the metabolism of specific drugs and therefore lessen their effect. Taking this herb with birth control pills, protease inhibitors, or immunosuppressant drugs is not recommended.

A dosage of 300 mg three times daily or 450 mg two times daily of a standardized extract of hypericin will give the best results.

Ginkgo is one of the oldest trees on Earth. The leaves of the ginkgo tree are very rich in antioxidants. The active ingredients are believed to help protect the brain and nervous system by scavenging free radicals. Another effect is mild thinning of the blood by decreasing platelet aggregation. This improves circulation throughout the body, and especially in the brain. Studies report that ginkgo improves short-term memory loss, depression, and cognitive function.

There have been numerous studies on the effects of ginkgo, some showing benefits among patients with dementia and Alzheimer's disease. The effects found were an increase in concentration, energy, and mood. A double-blind placebo-controlled study of 212 Alzheimer's patients treated for one year revealed significant improvement in cognition and social performance. Still, a recent study published in the *Journal of the American Medical Association* on normal patients aged sixty to eighty-two did not find significant benefits after four weeks of supplements. This study may have been too short to see an effect, or it could be that the effects are more apparent when a medical condition already exists.

If you are having memory problems, incorporate a supplement with ginkgo into your daily regimen. There are specific drug interactions, and since ginkgo has mild anticoagulant effects, it should not be used before surgery or with any anticoagulant medication. The recommended dosage is 60–120 mg two times daily. Combining ginkgo with ginseng can enhance the effects on concentration and cognition.

Brain Nutrients

Phosphatidylserine (PS) is the most abundant phospholipid in the brain. It is a component of cellular membranes and also found in the mitochondria. Taking PS on a regular basis will help restore brain and nerve function to normal. This supplement has been used to improve brain function, memory, and attention. Research studies have shown that phosphatidylserine increases the neurotransmitters dopamine, serotonin, acetylcholine, and norepinephrine.

Phosphatidylserine supplementation has been helpful for patients with Alzheimer's disease and attention deficit disorder10.

It is an essential nutrient that is present in many foods, but especially in soy. Most of the product available is from soy. The usual dosage is 100 mg three times daily. There are very few side effects to PS. If your memory is fading, try incorporating it into your regimen.

S-adenosyl-L-methionine (SAM-e) is a compound that is produced in the body, so it is not technically a vitamin. It combines the amino acid methionine and adenosine triphosphate (ATP), the energy molecule in the cell. In this combination, SAM-e becomes active in chemical reactions that affect many areas of the body. It contributes to the synthesis or activation of hormones, neurotransmitters, and proteins. Deficiencies of B_{12} and folate can cause lower-than-normal levels of SAM-e to be produced, leading to chronic health problems.

> **Mitochondria**
> *A mini organelle inside each cell made up of an accordion-shaped membrane where chemical reactions occur to produce energy from oxygen.*

SAM-e provides pain relief and reduces inflammation. Therefore it is useful for arthritis, fibromyalgia, and chronic pain. It also raises levels of the neurotransmitters serotonin, dopamine, and norepinephrine. When these levels are more balanced, anxiety and depression will resolve.

SAM-e should be used cautiously if you are taking antidepressant medication. Since it can increase levels of neurotransmitters, symptoms of agitation, anxiety, and tremors can occur. With some antidepressants, however, SAM-e improves the effectiveness of the medication. SAM-e can cause mania in those with bipolar disorder.

SAM-e protects the liver from damage from various drugs and is very helpful for liver disease. It is best to start with smaller dosages of 400 mg and work up to 1,600 mg daily. Side effects include nausea, vomiting, diarrhea, headache, and anxiety. If you are feeling depressed or anxious as your hormones falter, try taking SAM-e to boost your mood.

Acetyl-l-carnitine is one of the most extensively researched brain nutrients. It occurs naturally in the brain, increasing the energy of the brain cells and neurotransmitters, as well as repairing damage caused by stress and poor nutrition. In numerous research studies, acetyl-l-carnitine has been shown to reduce depression, increase recovery from strokes, and slow the progression of Alzheimer's disease. The only natural source of acetyl-l-carnitine is from the brains of animals that for numerous reasons are not recommended as a food. Therefore, the best option is to use a synthesized form derived from amino acids.

Acetyl-l-carnitine also appears to improve the function of the immune system. There are no side effects to this powerful nutrient, and its effects are often noticed within twenty minutes of taking it. Depending upon your medical condition, dosages of 700–3,000 mg are needed. Acteyl-l-carnitine works well when combined with other brain nutrients such as lipoic acid and phosphatidylserine.

SUMMARY OF MOOD BOOSTERS	
Pregnenolone	30–150 mg daily
DHEA	2.5–50 mg daily
Rhodiola	50–100 mg 2 times daily
St. John's wort	300 mg 3 times daily
Ginkgo	120–240 mg 2 times daily
SAM-e	400–1,600 mg daily
Phosphatidylserine	100 mg 3 times daily
Acetyl-l-carnitine	700–3,000 mg daily

CONCLUSION

Menopause is a process, not a disease. For a woman going through the process, education and understanding are the goals. By now, having read through this book, you should have many tools to help you make decisions for your health and well-being with your health practitioner.

The answer may be different for each woman, since we each carry our own genetic and lifetime issues, which will influence our choices. The key to a healthy life lies in individualizing your therapy based on your individual needs. Evaluate your need for hormones based on the symptoms you are experiencing and the other health issues you face. Weigh the potential risk of cancer, heart disease, Alzheimer's disease, or osteoporosis. Incorporate habits that will help maintain your health in this second half of your life with exercise, a healthy diet, supplements, and stress reduction techniques such as meditation or yoga.

Menopause is a time for magic. It is the time for that "menopausal zest" that Margaret Mead spoke of. A woman after menopause moves her creative focus from creating life to releasing that creative energy into society. There is also a grieving process that goes along with this as we lose our childbearing capacity and transition into a new chapter in life.

In ancient civilization, women were encouraged to find their rhythm and honored for the wisdom gained from menopause. As women in the twenty-first century, we must take that power back. It is an amazing journey as we walk together on this road to find the answer that is best for each of us.

I wish each of you blessings along your path.

REFERENCES

Arruzazabala, ML, et al. Comparative study of policosanol, aspirin and combination therapy policosanol-aspirin on platelet aggregation in healthy volunteers. *Pharmacol Res* 1997; 36(4):293–297.

Bass, FMS, et al. 13 betacarotene, B_6, folic acid, and zinc is associated with a lowered immune response and greater risk of developing cancer. *J Am Dietary Assoc,* 1995.

Cass, H. *Natural Highs.* New York: Avery Publications, 2002.

Editors of *Pharmacist's Letter* Natural Medicines Comprehensive Database, 2003.

Engelhart, MJ. Dietary intake of antioxidants and risk of Alzheimer's disease. *JAMA* 287(24):3223–3229.

Hannigan, B. *Brit J Biomed Sci,* 1994; 51:252–259.

Kronenberg F. Complementary and alternative medicine for menopausal symptoms: A review of randomized, controlled trials. *Ann Intern Med* Nov 19, 2002; 137(10): 805–813.

Lee, John R. *What your doctor may not tell you about breast cancer.* New York: Warner Books, 2003.

Pamer, E, et al. Predictors of longevity: A 25 year follow-up study. *Gerontologist* 1982; 6.

Saltman, PD, et al. The role of trace minerals in osteoporosis. *J Am Coll Nutr* 1993; 12:384–389.

Schnyder, G, et al. Effect of homocysteine-lowering therapy with folic acid, vitamin B_{12} and vitamin B_6 on clinical outcome after percutaneous coronary intervention. *JAMA* 2002; 288:973–979.

Swain, RA. Therapeutic uses of vitamin E in prevention of atherosclerosis. *Alt Med Rev* 1999; 4(6):414–423.

Vogel, JP. The death of anti-aging supplements. *Life Ext* March 2003.

Wald, D, et al. Homocysteine and cardiovascular disease: Evidence of causality from a meta-analysis. *BMJ* Jan 2003; 8:20–23.

RESOURCES

Love Potions, by C. M. Watson (published by Tarcher Putnam in New York, 2003).
For information regarding Dr. Watson's upcoming lectures, visit www.watsonwellness.org.

The Wisdom of Menopause by Christine Northrup.

What Your Doctor May Not Tell You About Menopause, by John Lee (published by Warner Books in New York).

North American Menopause Society
www.menopause.org.

International Academy of Compounding Pharmacists
www.healthy.net/professionals/compound.asp
 or 1-800-927-4227.

Laboratory Resources

Doctor's Data
P.O. Box 111
West Chicago, IL 60186
800-323-2784 (United States and Canada)
630-377-8139 (elsewhere)
www.doctorsdata.com

Great Smokies Diagnostic Laboratory
63 Zillicoa Street
Asheville, NC 28801
800-522-4762
www.gsdl.com

Metametrix
4855 Peachtree Industrial Boulevard
Norcross, GA 30092
770-446-5483
1-800-221-4640
www.metametrix.com

The Sedona Method
60 Tortilla Drive
Sedona, AZ 86336
928-282-3522
www.sedona.com

City of Hope
Cancer Genetics Education Program
1500 East Duarte Road
Duarte, CA 91010
1-800-826-4673
www.cityofhope.org/ccgp
For DNA cancer screening.

Periodicals

GreatLife Magazine
Consumer magazine with articles on vitamins, minerals, herbs, and foods.
Available for free at many health and natural food stores.

Let's Live Magazine
Consumer magazine with emphasis on the health benefits of vitamins, minerals, and herbs.

Customer service:
1-800-676-4333
P.O. Box 74908
Los Angeles, CA 90004
Subscriptions: 12 issues per year, $19.95 in the U.S.; $31.95 outside the U.S.

Physical Magazine
Magazine oriented to body builders and other serious athletes.

Customer service:
1-800-676-4333
P.O. Box 74908
Los Angeles, CA 90004
Subscriptions: 12 issues per year, $19.95 in the U.S.; $31.95 outside the U.S.

The Nutrition Reporter™ newsletter

Monthly newsletter that summarizes recent medical research on vitamins, minerals, and herbs.

Customer service:

P.O. Box 30246

Tucson, AZ 85751-0246

e-mail: jack@thenutritionreporter.com

www.nutritionreporter.com

Subscriptions: $26 per year (12 issues) in the U.S.; $32 U.S. or $48 CNC for Canada; $38 for other countries.

INDEX